The GOLDEN RATIΦ *within the* HUMAN FACE and BREAST

A PLASTIC SURGEON'S METHOD OF ANALYZING BEAUTY

Andrew J. Hayduke, M.D.

IVORY CROWN PRESS

Published by Ivory Crown Press - First Edition 2020
Beverly Hills, CA

ISBN 978-1-7359180-0-6 (pbk)

Library of Congress Control Number: 2020920454

The Golden Ratio Within the Human Face and Breast

To T. – the golden glitter in my life

and

To the thousands of patients who have entrusted themselves to me as their surgeon

TABLE OF CONTENTS

PREFACE

I've always been fascinated by the masters of art and the breathtaking beauty of their work. What perplexes me the most is why one particular piece of artwork—from a lifetime of excellent work—is singled out as an artist's masterpiece. To me, the masterpieces of world-renowned artists seem to possess something mystical concealed deep within them that radiates beauty, harmony, and proportion to an unusual degree. We can almost *feel* the beauty of the work. It's a surreal experience yet subconsciously palpable. Looking directly at an artist's original masterpiece with our own eyes, such as in the Louvre Museum in Paris or the Metropolitan Museum of Art in New York City, is the best way to experience this. Although it frequently goes unnoticed, I believe it's the underlying purity of form, proportion, and harmony within an artist's masterpiece that lays the foundation for its universally recognized brilliance. Needless to say, an artistic masterpiece has something truly special within it that's quite difficult to define. Something extraordinary exists within the work's composition that epitomizes beauty to the nth degree.

As a young child, I fondly remember attending after-school art classes that included formal hands-on instruction in both clay sculpture and drawing. I was always attracted to art, and creating realistic clay sculptures and drawings has been a part of my life to this day. I learned, from a very young age, that the process of creating realistic clay sculptures and drawings of the human form is founded upon certain rules and measurable proportions. I was taught that if I follow these general guidelines when creating realistic artwork of the human form, it's more likely that my work will ultimately look "right."

Science is another discipline that has always captivated me. Science yields order, logic, and sense from things that are complex and chaotic. Questions are answered, discoveries are made, and problems are solved based on concrete evidence and objective testing. Applying science to helping others—such as in the field of medicine—seemed to me a valiant pursuit. My love of science first led to an undergraduate bachelor's degree (summa cum laude) in the biological sciences. Medical school shortly followed and offered the opportunity for an in-depth, detailed study of my most beloved subject—human anatomy.

Gross human anatomy was a required class in the first year of medical school, and that experience will always hold a special place in my heart. I still remember the day when all of us young, eager medical students (all in our early 20s) tentatively walked into the medical school cadaver laboratory for the first time. It was definitely intimidating, but we pretended it wasn't. About 60 human cadavers were laid out on cold steel tables in the silent, eerie basement of the medical school. The intense smell of formaldehyde permeated the air. We meticulously dissected these human cadavers, inch by inch, almost daily. We were then mercilessly tested on the most minute intricacies of human anatomy by a team of expert PhD anatomists. As first-year medical students, we knew that academic excellence was expected from us, so we always strived to achieve an exam score of 100%. Although this experience was insanely competitive, intense, and grueling, it proved to be one of the most relevant classes of my life. I didn't realize it at the time, but that human anatomy class laid the foundation for my future both as a plastic surgeon and as an inventor.

After graduating from medical school, I chose plastic surgery for my postgraduate specialty training. I believe that plastic surgery provides the ideal blend of science and art. It's the best of both worlds, and no other surgical specialty offers that particular dynamic fusion. Plastic surgery allows me to express my passion for art, science, and human anatomic beauty all within a single surgical field—I simply couldn't ask for more. For me, plastic surgery was the obvious path to follow—not just as a career, but also as a life's passion.

I spent a total of seven years in surgical residency training after medical school graduation to learn the complex craft of plastic surgery. All of this formal training culminated in my eventual attainment of board certification by The American Board of Plastic Surgery. After all those long years of study and merciless testing, I finally achieved the stringent set of requirements to be legally referred to as a board certified plastic surgeon.

I've been practicing plastic surgery in Beverly Hills and Palm Springs, California, for my entire professional career. Beverly Hills is considered by many to be the global Mecca for cosmetic plastic surgery. I've had the pleasure of seeing patients in my private practice who are movie stars, rock stars, and internationally known celebrities. Needless to say, it never gets boring practicing plastic surgery in sunny Southern California, where maintaining an attractive physical appearance always seems to be a priority. The standards are high for the quality of work that I'm expected to produce, and I enjoy that challenge.

Having been in the clinical practice of plastic surgery since 2002, I've performed thousands of plastic surgery procedures on both the face and breasts. All these years of clinical practice served to expose both the strengths and weaknesses of plastic surgery as a surgical subspecialty. I eventually discovered that one of the shortcomings in the field of modern plastic surgery is the lack of a universal, objective, measurement-based method for assessing beauty within the human face and breasts.

It's common for plastic surgeons to hear new patients ask, "Doctor, what do you think I should do?" Although patients don't realize it, plastic surgeons frequently make educated guesses about many issues during the presurgical decision-making process. For example, surgeons might ask themselves: How large of a chin implant should I use? How high should I raise the eyebrows with browlift surgery for this patient's unique face? What size breast implants would best fit this particular patient's body frame? How high should the nipple be raised in this patient with severe breast droop (ptosis)? To me, answering these types of questions with a casual educated-guess approach seems akin to creating artwork with no true measurement-based foundation or proportional guidelines. Although some crude guidelines for plastic surgeons do indeed exist, they're certainly not enough. I felt that something within the field of plastic surgery was lacking, and the methods for assessing physical beauty desperately needed to be improved upon.

In most cases, invention is born of necessity. First and foremost, I believe there's a need for something better than just an educated guess for patients seeking facial or breast plastic surgery of the highest caliber. After all, when I was still a young child learning the fundamentals of realistic clay sculpture and drawing of the human form, certain underlying guidelines were always emphasized. I believe it's also reasonable to create some type of objective measurable guidelines for plastic surgery and for the assessment of beauty and proportion within human anatomy.

The relevance of testing for beauty in human anatomy extends far beyond plastic surgery. Endeavors such as modeling, acting, beauty pageant competition, and other pursuits where physical appearance is critical to success can benefit from an objective analysis of human physical beauty. In some cases, casting agents and Hollywood producers could benefit from an additional objective tool to help them discover actors with the "right" look—especially if the role requires physical beauty.

In this brief treatise, I provide an all-access, backstage pass to the clinical analysis methodologies I use in my plastic surgery practice. I describe the specific methods and tests I currently apply when analyzing beauty within the human face and breasts, an endeavor I usually perform secretly. My descriptions of these tests are quite detailed, to the point that they may occasionally seem geared more toward a practicing plastic surgeon rather than the general reader. However, nonphysician readers who would enjoy a detailed, behind-the-scenes sneak peek at how a Beverly Hills plastic surgeon truly evaluates his patient's anatomic beauty (or lack thereof) may find the descriptions enlightening.

I also explore the concept of human beauty itself being an objective quality rather than a mere subjective opinion. I describe various fascinating methodologies and components of human physical beauty that have been proposed over the years by other talented research scientists. I don't contend that my own beauty analysis methods provide the sole explanation for something as complex as human physical beauty. I hope, however, that my work at least contributes some valuable insight into understanding the objective and measurable components of human physical beauty.

CHAPTER 1

OBJECTIVITY AND SCIENCE WITHIN BEAUTY

Merging of Philosophy, Art, and Mathematics

What exactly is physical beauty? Is it found in the architectural structure of the Parthenon in Greece? Do we find it in the high cheekbones, enchanting eyes, and stunning facial features of the latest magazine cover model, or is it found in nature in the arrangement of petals within a flower or the gently winding spirals of a nautilus seashell? Do we *feel* beauty, or do we *see* beauty?

Formally, beauty is defined as "the quality or aggregate of qualities in a person or thing that gives pleasure to the senses or pleasurably exalts the mind or spirit."[1] This is a definition that has oscillated beyond measure. The rhetoric within modern-day media and within our current society has convinced most of us—for better or worse—that physical beauty isn't bound by this definition. It seems we're currently expected to believe that physical beauty is a largely subjective thing—but is it really? Self-help gurus often take liberty to say that *everyone* is beautiful, while others dismiss beauty as a trivial, superficial concern. We're all acquainted with the old adage "Beauty is in the eye of the beholder." We carelessly toss the term around wherever we please, abandoning the objective implications of beauty's actual definition, which calls for a specific aggregate of qualities within a person or thing. Though we can—and likely will—continue to stretch the meaning of beauty to suit our needs, no amount of twisting, turning, or bending circumvents the necessity to confront and contemplate the complexities of human physical beauty.

When I personally see something that appears beautiful to me, I sense something within that physical object that gives me immediate pleasure. Something just simply seems right about it, summoning my immediate admiration for no obvious tangible reason. Why something appears physically beautiful is a fascinating mystery, which we often dismiss by our knee-jerk reaction of defining beauty as purely subjective. I suggest there may be something more, something measurable and quantifiable, hidden deep within a physical object or even within a person's anatomy that can help explain why it radiates beauty. I suggest that physical beauty, including human anatomic beauty, is largely an objective quality rather than a mere subjective opinion.

Beauty is a complex subject. In fact, an entire branch of philosophy is dedicated to understanding it. Aesthetics is defined as "a branch of philosophy dealing with the nature of beauty, art, and taste and with the creation and appreciation of beauty."[2] The word *aesthetics* is derived from the Greek word *aisthētikos,* meaning "of sense perception."[2] Based on the qualities and physical features of an object (or person), we all have a certain response when we view it. The reaction we have to an object's physical appearance, based upon our perception of the object, is generally referred to as an "aesthetic response."[3]

In the most basic sense, how we perceive an object involves both the physical elements within that object and the adherence of the object's physical elements to certain principles. "Physical elements" refer to the parts that make up the object. The "principles" comprise the relationships among those parts—e.g., unity, balance, proportion. When we view the physical appearance of certain objects or people, this may elicit in us a favorable aesthetic response, and we immediately label these objects or people as physically beautiful.

Some researchers believe that nonconscious cognitive-processing algorithms (i.e., internal processing algorithms) automatically dictate our aesthetic response to physical objects.[4,5] Perhaps, as human beings, we're all somehow similarly wired to perceive physical beauty within another person or object. Our aesthetic response is believed to be immediate, automatic, and guided by nonconscious cognitive-processing algorithms that we simply don't have access to or conscious control of. I will try to solve the mystery of what, specifically, within the viewed object guides those cognitive-processing algorithms that tell us to automatically label something or someone as physically "beautiful."

We can't earnestly place beauty in a box labeled "to each their own" and release ourselves from the uncomfortable acknowledgment that *some* things and *some* people may not be physically beautiful. As a result of our current society's efforts to democratize the term, we seem to have lost sight of beauty's immense significance in our everyday lives. The consequences of our physical appearance began to affect our lives from the time we took our first breath. Research studies have shown that infants who are physically attractive are treated preferentially by caregivers. This includes increased attention given to physically beautiful newborns by neonatal nurses and better treatment of attractive infants by their very own mothers.[6,7,8,9,10,11,12,13,14] Physical appearance also affected how we were treated and what was expected from us in preschool, elementary school, high-school, and college—both by well-intentioned teachers and our peers.[15,16,17,18,19,20,21,22,23,24,25] Physical appearance affects our adult social interactions (dating behaviors), careers, financial success, marriage, and even how supposedly impartial judges and juries rule for or against us in the courtroom.[26,27,28,29,30,31,32,33,34,35,36,37,38,39] There's no doubt that physical beauty is a massive, commanding force that informs small and large decisions on micro- and macrocosmic scales. It's a market-steering notion that feeds entire industries and employs millions of people.

Beauty is deeply enmeshed in the entire history and development of mankind, yet efforts to obscure its interpretation and significance are ceaseless. Physical beauty, or lack thereof, *always was* and *always will be* a significant factor in our lives. Whether we realize it or not is a different story. Accepting the cold reality that physical beauty is not common and not possessed by all is indeed a difficult pill to swallow.

Consider architects and urban planners, who design entire cities, neighborhoods, communities, individual homes, and, ultimately, create the backdrop of our lives. Ponder the job of interior decorators, who are hired to arrange a number of components in a very specific way to create satisfying and visually appealing spaces in which we live and work. They strive to arrange objects at very precise distances, locations, and in appropriate proportions to create work that's considered aesthetically beautiful. Their goal is to create a positive aesthetic response. Some are very successful at what they do, and some are not.

What this all means is that, in positions that involve aesthetic decision making, "good" and "bad" are values that exist. Some architectural designs are considered amazing aesthetic achievements that are universally admired by architectural experts, while other designs are considered outright unattractive disasters. Similarly, some works of fine art are so beautiful that they're housed in the Louvre in France and visited by millions of tourists from around the world. Other works of art lack such beauty and sit sadly unsold at neighborhood yard sales or discount resale shops. According to Forbes, the beautiful faces of the highest-paid fashion models can earn them well over $20 million per year.[40] The rest of us "normal," everyday people probably weren't lucky enough to hit the same genetic jackpot of physical beauty. Our physical appearance may have proven to be a significant detriment to our personal relationships, education, employment, financial success, and many other aspects of our lives. The cold reality is some things possess physical beauty and some things simply do not.

Why, then, is modern society's view of beauty drenched in subjectivity when it comes to the way we look? Less delicately, why do we pretend that human physical beauty can't be objectively measured? In what follows, I'll discuss some of the illuminating findings of researchers who've conducted studies to demystify the concept of human physical beauty. Human physical beauty has been widely investigated using the scientific method throughout the last century. As we'll discover, the findings point to a universally comparable value measure of human physical attractiveness and beauty. It seems there *is* an understanding of beauty as a concept with a scope far greater than that of the beholder. But what's the force that steers where the needle falls? What is it within an object's appearance that causes us to consider it physically beautiful? Why are we rarely alone in what or whom we consider to be physically beautiful? More specifically, is physical beauty a subjective or an objective thing?

Antiquity's Perspective on Objective Beauty

To fully understand beauty and all of its intricacies, we must go back to the first documented explorations and meditations on beauty. The works of prolific philosophers, mathematical discoveries, and important pieces of history all inform our understanding of beauty's essential definition as a quality or qualities that give "pleasure to the senses or pleasurably exalt the mind or spirit."[1] We'll examine whether these qualities are objective or merely a subjective opinion. Also, is beauty somehow related to mathematical harmony and proportion of the individual physical elements that make up that object?

The logical place to begin to answer these questions is to explore the beliefs of the great philosophers of antiquity regarding aesthetics and beauty. Plato said, "There are things which are beautiful always and by themselves."[41] This perspective of beauty has been referred to as aesthetic objectivity. Plato didn't feel that the personal opinion of the beholder had anything to do with beauty. Beauty, to Plato, was an objective thing that existed within the object itself rather than as an external subjective opinion about the object. Aristotle said, "To be beautiful, a living creature, and every whole made up of parts, must … present a certain order in its arrangement of parts."[42] With regard to mathematics within beauty, Aristotle said, "The chief forms of beauty are order and symmetry and definiteness, which the mathematical sciences demonstrate in a special degree."[43]

One of the earliest attempts to objectively quantify beauty can be traced to the ancient Greeks. Many believe that the great Greek philosopher and mathematician Pythagoras of Samos (570–495 BC) provided the earliest accounts relating beauty with ratios, mathematical relationships, proportions, and harmony. Pythagoreans (followers of Pythagoras) believed that beauty had its origins in harmony, order, proportions, measurements, and numbers. Although perhaps a bit harsh, the Pythagoreans believed that "order and proportion are beautiful and useful, while disorder and lack of proportion are ugly and useless."[44] The views of the Pythagoreans support the premise that beauty is largely objective. Plato agreed with the Pythagoreans, stating, "Nothing which is beautiful is without proportion."[45] Plato's beliefs solidified the notion of aesthetic objectivity for several millennia that followed.

Pythagoras related beauty with mathematics and proportions, albeit it in the world of music and astronomy. The philosophical concept of "Harmony of the Spheres" (*Musica universalis*) was born, which contended that the sun, moon, and planets each produce unique tones based on their orbits and revolutions. Pythagoras also believed that certain mathematical ratios existed between the intervals of beautiful harmonious sounds.

The concept of beauty being related to mathematics, proportions, and ratios seems to have its origins in the mind of this legendary Greek philosopher. His work clearly supported the notion that beauty is objective and that there are quantifiable reasons for beauty. Some believe that Pythagoras and his followers discovered the mathematical ratio of 1.0:1.618 to be quintessential to beauty and attractive proportion. (This ratio, 1.0:1.618, would later be formally named the "divine proportion," but not until about 1500 AD.)

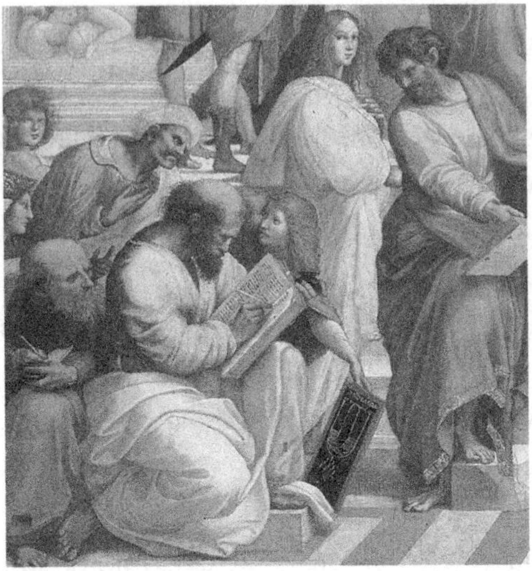

Figure 1. *The School of Athens* (detail of fresco) by Raphael (c. 1509–1511). This image is cropped on Pythagoras writing down his ideas while surrounded by a group of curious onlookers.

The ancient Greeks are perhaps best known for creating artistic work that depicts the classic, ideal male form. Phideas, a renowned Greek sculptor, was commissioned to create the *Statue of Zeus at Olympia*. This work depicts the Greek god Zeus as a lean, muscular, athletic male with minimal body fat. Phideas was likely influenced by the athletic build of male athletes competing in the Olympic games taking place at that time. After all, the true purpose of the Olympic games during the ancient Greek period was to honor Zeus. In addition, Phideas created *Athena Parthenos*, an enormous statue of the stunning Greek goddess Athena that resided in the Parthenon (Figure 2). By modern standards, however, she'd be considered overweight and certainly not athletic.

Many believe that Phideas used the "divine proportion" of 1.0:1.618 (golden ratio) to guide the creation of his many outstanding works of sculptural beauty. The Greek letter phi (upper case ϕ or lower case φ) is commonly used to symbolize the golden ratio in mathematics. The phi symbol was chosen to pay homage to the name Phideas (Φειδιας in Ancient Greek).

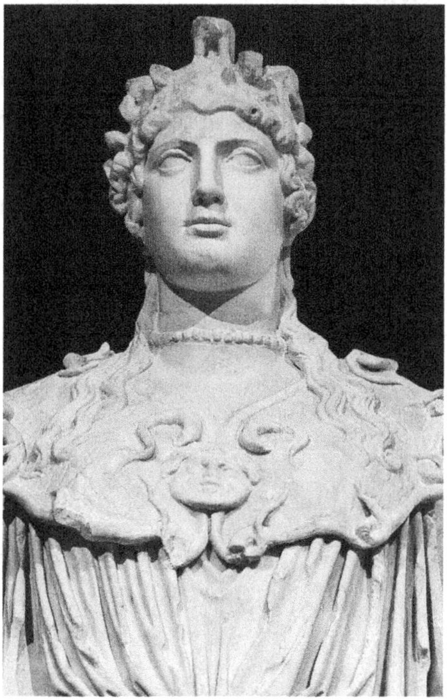

Figure 2. *Athena Parthenos* by Phideas, second-century AD Roman copy.

Polycleitus was another Greek sculptor who had a major influence on Western ideas of human physical beauty. He lived in the same time period as Phideas. His most famous sculptural work is the male nude sculpture *Doryphoros* ("Spear Bearer"), also referred to as *Canon* (Figure 3). Unlike Phideas, Polycleitus actually provided explanations and rules for creating beautiful, realistic proportions in human sculpture in his famous written work, *Canon of Polycleitus*. In this work, Polycleitus provided a set of guidelines (rules) for the proper harmonious proportions of the human body based on the individual parts of the whole. This was achieved, for example, by relating the finger to the palm, the palm to the forearm, the forearm to the upper arm, and so forth. Using this particular set of rules, Polycleitus was said to have created his masterpiece sculpture *Doryphoros* (Figure 3). Polycleitus provided clear, written, objective guidelines for beauty within the human form.

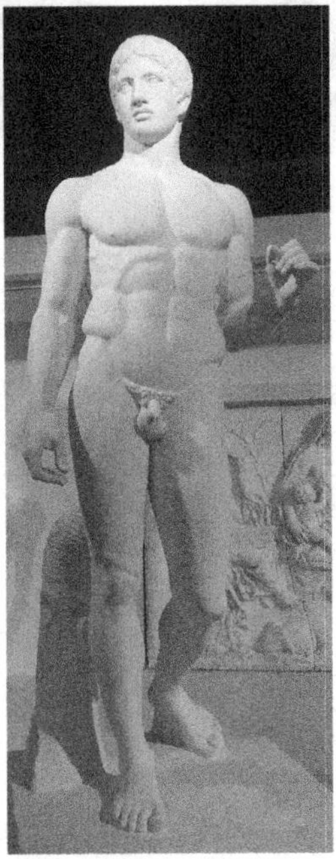

Figure 3. *Doryphoros* ("Spear Bearer") by Polycleitus, plaster cast of a first-century AD Roman copy.

Summetria is an ancient Greek word for the concept that proper proportion is absolutely essential for beauty. Polycleitus generally receives credit for creating the concept that *summetria* lies at the core of all things pleasing to the human eye. The concept of objectivity within beauty was being solidified by attempting to unlock the underlying reasons for beauty based upon objective measurement and proportion.

The Romans further embraced the idea of objectivity and mathematical proportions in beauty. Vitruvius Pollio was a legendary Roman architect and military engineer. He's most famous for creating a ten-volume work on architecture called *De architectura* for the Roman emperor Caesar Augustus. Surprisingly, in chapter one of book three of *De architectura*, Vitruvius describes the proper architectural design of a temple as it relates to the proper proportions of a human body and face. This brilliant architect's written description of human body proportions is an invaluable addition to the understanding of human beauty. It may seem surprising that it came from the mind of an architect, but it provides a set of firm guidelines or rules (canons) for what creates an attractive human appearance. Vitruvius writes:

> If we take the height of the face itself, the distance from the bottom of the chin to the underside of the nostrils is one third of it; the nose from the underside of the nostrils to a line between the eyebrows is the same; from there to the lowest roots of the hair is also a third, comprising the forehead.[46]

Later in the chapter, Vitruvius describes the body as it relates to the length of a human foot: "The length of the foot is one sixth of the height of the body; of the forearm, one fourth; and the breadth of the breast is also one fourth."[46]

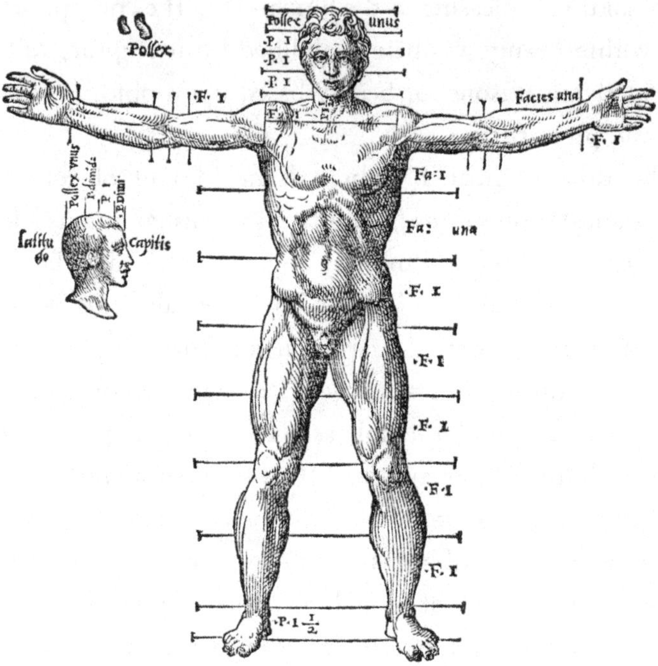

Figure 4. Illustration from *De architectura libri decem*, originally written by Vitruvius Pollio (c. 30–15 BC). This illustration is from an edition published by Daniele Barbaro (1567).

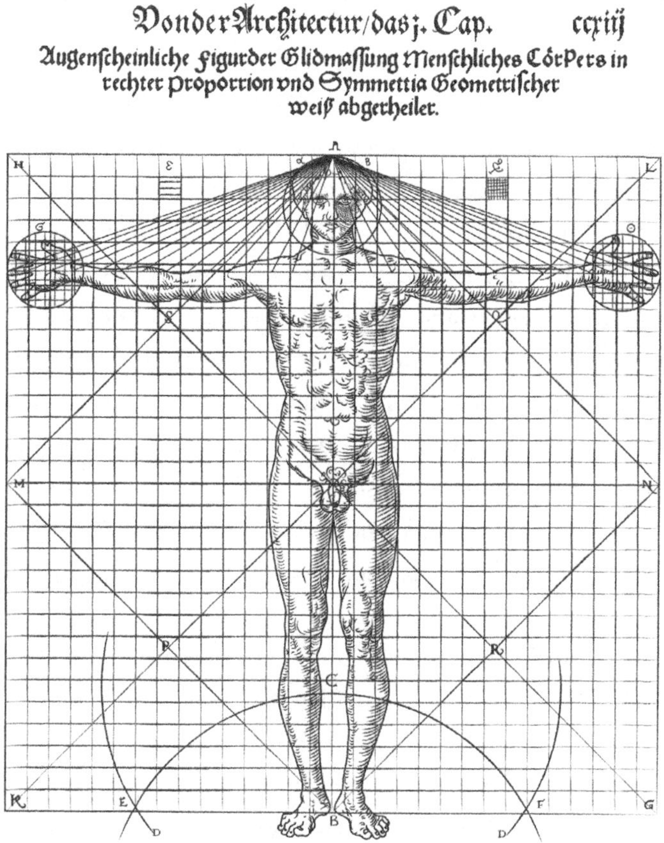

Figure 5. *Human Proportion Figure* (*Menschliche Proportionsfigur*) by Walther Hermann Ryff (1575). This illustration is based on Vitruvius Pollio's work.

Based upon prior work of the ancient Greeks, Plato, and various mathematicians, Vitruvius also discussed whether the number ten or the number six should be considered the "perfect number" as it relates to harmonious structure and proportional relationships within a beautiful human form.

Beauty's Evolution during the Renaissance Period

Luca Pacioli was a brilliant Italian mathematician and writer during the Renaissance period (approximately 1300–1600 AD). He wrote a famous work on mathematics called *De devina Proportione.* This work describes the golden ratio as it relates to architecture, geometry, and art. To illustrate his book, Pacioli hired Leonardo da Vinci.

The Renaissance period was known as an era of rebirth characterized by renewed and fervent interest in classical Greek and Roman philosophy, art, and literature. This period represents the transition from medieval times to modern times. Most Renaissance writers believed that beauty is objective. Leon Battista Alberti, a prominent Renaissance philosopher, said, "According to my convictions, there are certain principles, values, and rules in each art and science. He who finds them and carefully applies them, will achieve his aims beautifully."[47]

Leonardo da Vinci (1452–1519) epitomized the definition of a "Renaissance man." He's considered by some to be possibly the greatest genius to have ever lived. His diversity of talent spanned an unprecedented variety of fields, including painting, human anatomy, mathematics, engineering, science, literature, astronomy, geology, and cartography. During his training as an artist, he was allowed to dissect human corpses at several hospitals throughout Italy. Da Vinci created amazingly detailed sketches, drawings, and notes on human anatomy.

One of da Vinci's most famous works is *Vitruvian Man*, created in honor of Vitruvius Pollio (Figure 6). Leonardo da Vinci used the proportions of the human male described by Vitruvius Pollio to create this drawing—with a few minor modifications based on his own study of human anatomy. It depicts a man with arms and legs spread apart within a circle as well as within a square.

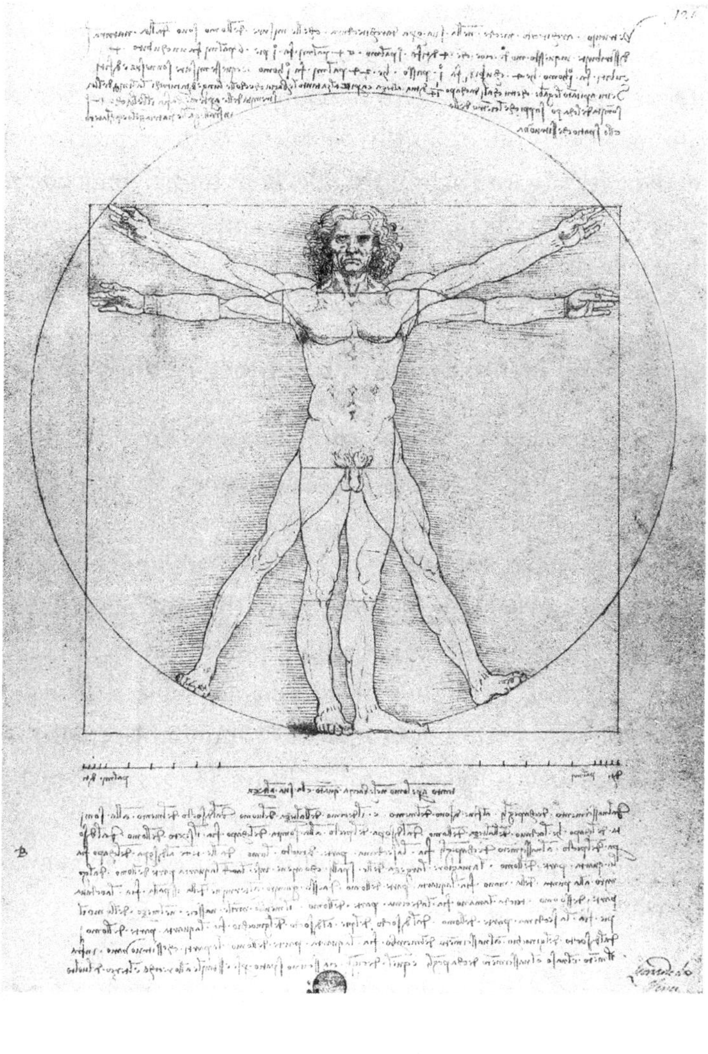

Figure 6. *Vitruvian Man* by Leonardo da Vinci (c. 1490).

Leonardo's prior collaboration with mathematician Luca Pacioli on *De devina Proportione,* combined with his own advanced knowledge of human anatomy, led some to speculate that Leonardo may have incorporated the golden ratio into several of his later masterpieces. These include legendary paintings such as *The Last Supper* and *Mona Lisa*. Perhaps the mind of this unique genius was able to incorporate all of his diverse talents with his previous study of mathematics (with Pacioli) to unlock an underlying code or set of rules to follow when attempting to express human beauty and aesthetically pleasing, harmonious proportion in art.

The Shift from an Objective to a Subjective View of Beauty

With an understanding of the early conceptualization of beauty and its ties to objective mathematical theories, we now shift our lens to the mechanics of beauty's subjective baptism and take stock of how the foundation given to us by these early pioneers may call into question how we view beauty today. The post-Renaissance period marked a major shift in the philosophical view of beauty from a largely objective quality to a predominantly subjective one.

The objective notion of beauty was commonplace until David Hume's essay "On the Standard of Taste" (1757) reignited a reconsideration of beauty's nature. The Scottish philosopher wrote, "Beauty is no quality in things themselves: it exists merely in the mind which contemplates them."[48] Over the last couple of centuries, Hume's reassessment has inspired numerous texts on the matter. Immanuel Kant, an influential German philosopher, furthered the belief that no specific objective property within a thing makes it beautiful. Kant's *Critique of Judgment* (*Kritik der Urteilskraft*), published in 1790, deeply explored aesthetics. Kant propagated the belief that judgments of beauty are "subjectively grounded."[49]

Ever since the work of Hume and Kant, subjective notions of beauty seem to have dominated modern thought. These beliefs persist to this very day and have even trickled down into modern axioms. The phrase "eye of the beholder" lurks between the pages of bestsellers—books that you ought to never "judge by their covers"—and remember, "beauty is only skin-deep." These cultural maxims have become so intrinsic to our modern-day social fabric that it would seem almost distasteful to call them into question—but I do.

Evidence from contemporary research indicates that these sayings are more akin to myths than fact. Mantras that reject the objective properties of beauty may be a crutch or coping mechanism for those who believe they can't meet certain ideals. Arguably, there's a necessity for these maxims, as beauty can and *does* affect the way we experience life, but whether that's fair or not is a separate debate altogether.

Modern Research Supports the Objective Nature of Physical Beauty

Modern sophisticated technology allows for a deeper insight into the complexities of physical beauty and whether it has a significant objective component. We now have the luxury of advanced technologies that couldn't even be imagined a mere 100 years ago, much less by the key influential proponents of a subjective view of beauty such as Hume and Kant in the 1700s. For example, technology now allows us to obtain a truly objective evaluation of human brain activity based on blood-flow patterns to specific areas of the brain. Functional magnetic resonance imaging (fMRI) objectively measures and documents which areas of the human brain experience the most blood flow in real time while a person is actively doing a specific task or looking at certain images (stimuli). The exact location of greatest brain activity as a result of any given stimulus can be localized to within a few millimeters.

In one recent study, a research team led by Di Dio modified a photographic image of the classic sculpture of *Doryphoros* to create a total of three versions of this sculpture. One of the versions depicted the sculpture with the attractive 1.0:1.618 ratio of the sculpture's original proportions. The other two images violated this ratio to create two "ugly" versions of this same nude sculpture using ratios of 1.0:1.36 and 1.0:1.74. Reviewers were then asked to look at these images while fMRI scans of their brains were simultaneously performed.

Di Dio et al. concluded:

> The main question we addressed in the present study was whether there is an objective beauty, i.e., if objective parameters intrinsic to works of art are able to elicit a specific neural pattern underlying the sense of beauty in the observer. Our results gave a positive answer to this question. The presence of a specific parameter (the golden ratio) in the stimuli we presented determined brain activations different to those where this parameter was violated.[50]

Di Dio et al. found evidence for an objective, biological basis of the experience of physical beauty. He also found that the region of the brain that showed the most activity on fMRI when people looked at the image of the beautiful sculpture incorporating the *golden ratio* was the anterior insula. The insula is a region of the human brain that also happens to be linked to sexual orgasm and emotion.

In a different study, Shen evaluated the fMRI results of the brain responses of 41 adults who looked at images of human faces with altered facial proportions. The facial proportions were those found in a previous study to be related to facial attractiveness. Shen concluded, "Our results indicate that some specific facial ratios play important roles in determining the facial attractiveness. This finding provides us additional neurophysiological evidence for the suggestion that attractive faces follow optimum facial proportions."[51] The specific parts of the brain where facial attractiveness seemed to show "significant linear effects" were the postcentral gyrus, caudate nucleus, and bilateral inferior frontal gyrus.

Nedeljkovic investigated whether there is a difference in the proportions of anonymous female faces versus the faces of attractive, female celebrities. He compared the facial proportions of 83 anonymous University of Belgrade female students, aged 22 to 28, with 24 female celebrity faces. His study demonstrated significant differences in facial-proportion measurements between the anonymous group and the celebrity group. He also found that the facial measurements within the celebrity group all seemed to conform to certain proportions.[52]

Other researchers compared the facial features of attractive television actresses with the faces of normal, healthy females. They concluded that "facial characteristics of the beautiful women were significantly different from the characteristics of the normal women."[53] They also found that the facial characteristics of the beautiful actresses were more "uniform" in appearance with less variation. This study meticulously analyzed several angles, ratios, linear distances, and volumes within the studied faces. These studies seem to agree that objective, measurable qualities within the facial features of beautiful (attractive) celebrity faces were indeed different from those found in the faces of ordinary people who were not involved in the entertainment industry.

Many studies have found evidence of objective, measurable components within attractive human faces. A study of 50 females between the ages 18 and 20 found that certain facial profile proportions received higher aesthetic scores only if they were close to the golden ratio.[54] The facial profiles that received the lower aesthetic scores by the 20 judges did not have proportions close to the golden ratio. Another study analyzed the facial-feature proportions of 90 beautiful magazine-cover models compared with 34 "non-attractive" individuals chosen from a group of orthodontic patients. This study concluded that the attractive cover models had facial proportions closer to the golden ratio as compared with the non-attractive faces. The author concluded that "facial beauty is measurable to some degree."[55]

If my personal belief is true—that human physical beauty is founded on objective criteria (such as measurements between human anatomical features)—there should be evidence of cross-cultural and cross-ethnic agreement regarding who is physically beautiful. Significant research has indeed been done in this area. The attractiveness judgments of white Scots and black South Africans were tested for both same- and other-ethnicity faces. The results showed there was agreement between the judgments of both white Scots and black South Africans on which faces were attractive. The authors stated, "These results provide further evidence of the universality of facial attractiveness preferences."[56]

Another study asked native Asians, Hispanics and white Americans to judge photographic images of Asian, Hispanic, black, and white women for attractiveness. The results showed a strong agreement between the ethnic groups for judgments regarding attractiveness (correlation coefficient $r = .93$).[57]

Cross-cultural researchers asked judges from two dramatically different cultures to rate facial traits, including physical attractiveness, of individuals within and outside their own culture. One group of judges used in this study were Tsimane people from the Bolivian rainforest. The villages where the Tsimane people currently live don't have electricity or running water. The other group of judges were from the industrialized United States. The results showed that, despite the extreme isolation of the Tsimane people within a rainforest, "Tsimane as well as U.S. judges showed within-culture agreement in impressions of attractiveness ... of own-culture faces." In addition, the study found that "both groups also showed within-culture agreement for impressions of other-culture faces."[58] The researchers went on to say that they found between-culture agreement for faces (especially for Tsimane faces) and that the cross-cultural similarities in trait impressions from the two groups of judges support a "universal mechanism."

In scientific research, a meta-analysis is a study that combines the results of several previous, independent studies on the exact same research topic. The conclusions of the statistical analysis derived from a large meta-analysis are much more meaningful (with more statistical power) than the conclusions of just one individual research study. Langlois et al. published a meta-analysis that looked at articles and references from a nearly 70-year span of research on "objectively rated facial attractiveness." This study included an initial sample of over 1,800 empirical articles. Langlois et al. concluded that both within and across cultures, raters agreed on who is and is not attractive. The researchers went on to say:

> Both our cross-cultural and cross-ethnic agreement-effect sizes are more than double the size necessary

> to be considered large, suggesting a possibly universal standard by which attractiveness is judged. These analyses seriously question the common assumption that attractiveness ratings are culturally unique and merely represent media-induced standards.[59]

Evidence from all this scientific research, including direct fMRI studies of human brain activity, points to objectivity and universal qualities as the true foundation of human physical beauty. Naturally, these scientific findings might make some of us a little uncomfortable. If human physical beauty is based largely on objective and measurable qualities, then some of us *will* and some of us *will not* possess those specific qualities. Physical beauty is representative of an unfair inequality among humans—an inequality that was genetically bestowed upon us (in our DNA) at the time we were conceived. Because of current society's focus on political correctness, this cruel inequality of Nature has made even the mere suggestion of objectivity within human physical beauty a kind of taboo. Nowadays, it seems almost rude to suggest such a preposterous idea as aesthetic objectivity. Regardless of what current society expects us to believe, physical beauty (or lack thereof) is indeed a major entity working in the shadows of our lives that we all know is there yet are usually unwilling to openly admit. Perhaps it's a comfortable coping mechanism for us to politely pretend that human physical beauty is a trivial part of our lives that's largely based on the mere opinion of the observer.

Although we certainly haven't solved beauty's conundrum, hopefully this brief exploration of aesthetics sheds some light on the foundations of the concept and the way in which our understanding of it has evolved. Aesthetic subjectivity is, for the most part and unfortunately, accepted in our society's current views on beauty. I suggest, however, that we reconsider the currently fashionable philosophical viewpoint of a subjective assessment of physical beauty and instead embrace the concept of objectivity in aesthetics. I suggest we give more weight to both modern sophisticated research and to the ideas of some of the greatest minds in history—Plato, Aristotle, Pythagoras, Polycleitus, Vitruvius, Pacioli, and Leonardo da Vinci. Following the path directed by these ancient thinkers and by the conclusions of a substantial body of contemporary scientific research, I contend that beauty isn't simply in the eye of the beholder. I believe the majority of qualities that characterize human physical beauty are objective, universal, and clinically measurable. One such measurable quality, famously enmeshed within physical beauty and attractive proportion, exists within the mathematical relationship known as the golden ratio.

CHAPTER 2

ALL THAT GLITTERS IS GOLD

Fundamentals of the Golden Ratio

My method of analyzing the human face and breasts for beauty is rooted in golden ratio relationships. The first step to understanding the logic of my method is to explore the fundamentals of the renowned golden ratio, golden rectangle, and golden spiral.

The golden ratio (also known as the *divine proportion*, *divine section*, *golden number*, and *golden mean*) is thought to be involved in many harmonious relationships within mathematics, geometry, art, music, nature, and architecture. The golden ratio can be expressed as the mathematical ratio of 1.618:1.0. Many people, including myself, believe that the presence of a golden ratio relationship within an object serves as the core underlying foundation for a beautiful, balanced, proportional, and attractive appearance of that particular object. Simply put, a physical object just seems to look "right" if golden ratio relationships exist within the individual components of that particular object.

The Golden Ratio in Graphic Arts

We don't need to look any farther than the eye-catching logos of successful businesses for modern-day examples of the use of the golden ratio. Contemporary graphic artists strategically use golden ratio relationships in the designs of many well-known company logos. We, as consumers, are completely unaware of this fact, but successful graphic artists and advertisers are keenly aware that golden ratio visual relationships are particularly attractive to the human eye. The visual appeal of the logo of a company is extremely important to the company's overall image. It serves as the visual basis of the brand's memory recall for potential and existing customers–which ultimately translates into sales (i.e., money and profits). The importance of the visual symbol that represents a brand is reflected by the fact that many large companies spend a mind-boggling amount of money on logo designs, redesigns, and rebranding. For example, the Pepsi logo redesign cost $1 million, the British Broadcasting Company (BBC) logo redesign and rebranding cost $1.8 million, and the British Petroleum rebranding and logo redesign cost $211 million.[1]

Figure 7 shows how several well-known global companies have ingeniously incorporated the golden ratio into their logos.

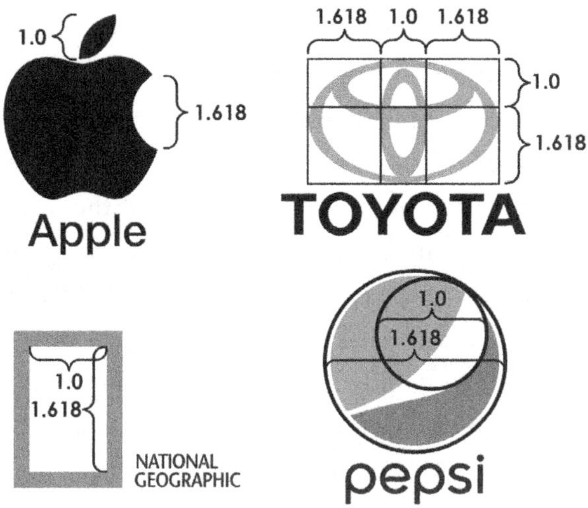

Figure 7. Golden ratio relationships hidden within the design of several famous logos (logos displayed are registered trademarks of their respective companies).

The Golden Ratio in Architecture

Golden ratio relationships can also be found in architecture. Egyptian Old Kingdom–era architecture includes one of the most famous ancient examples of the apparent use of the golden ratio in a structure. The Great Pyramid of Giza is one of the Seven Wonders of the Ancient World. This pyramid was created from about 2.3 million stone blocks each weighing approximately 2.5 tons.[2] Egyptian pyramids were built as tombs for pharaohs (kings) and were fully equipped with everything the pharaohs would need for their afterlives. Some believe that the pyramids' sides were angled to help the pharaoh's soul ascend to heaven.

As shown in Figure 8, Kepler triangles can be drawn within the Great Pyramid of Giza. One of the angled sides of the pyramid contains the triangle's hypotenuse (the longest side of a right triangle located opposite the right angle). The second side is created by dropping a vertical line from the triangle's apex to a point on its floor. The third side runs from that point to the side of the pyramid containing the hypotenuse. The ratio of the side of the Kepler triangle on the pyramid's floor and of its hypotenuse reduces to the golden ratio. The presence of this golden ratio relationship within the Great Pyramid of Giza imparts a strong sense of harmony and balance. Due to its undeniably sound architectural construction, the Great Pyramid of Giza holds the distinction of being the only member of the Seven Wonders of the Ancient World that still remains standing to this day.

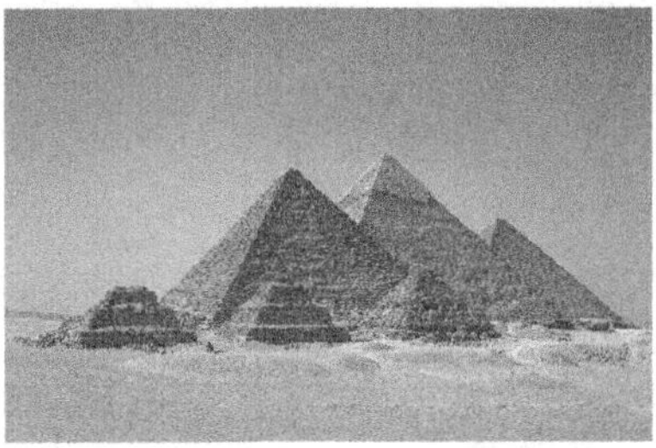

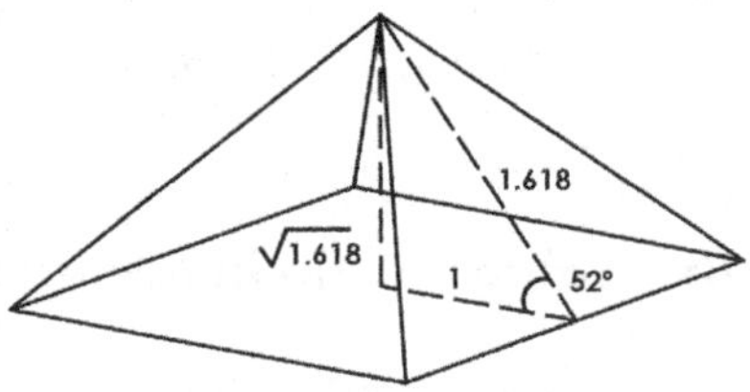

Figure 8. Left: The Giza pyramid complex in Egypt (c. 2580–2560 BC). Right: The Kepler triangle (illustrated with dashed lines) is a right triangle whose short side and hypotenuse lengths form a ratio that reduces to 1.0:1.618. Architecturally, the Great Pyramid of Giza (the largest pyramid in the image above) is a "golden pyramid" due to its inclusion of the Kepler triangle.

The Parthenon in Athens (c. 432 BC) is a temple dedicated to the goddess Athena. It's considered a Greek architectural masterpiece. The sculptor Phidias created an ivory and gold statue of Athena for the interior and was also involved in the Parthenon's overall architecture.[3] Several golden ratio relationships seem to be hidden within the Parthenon's structural design (Figure 9). It's very likely that this is due to the influence and guidance of Phidias.

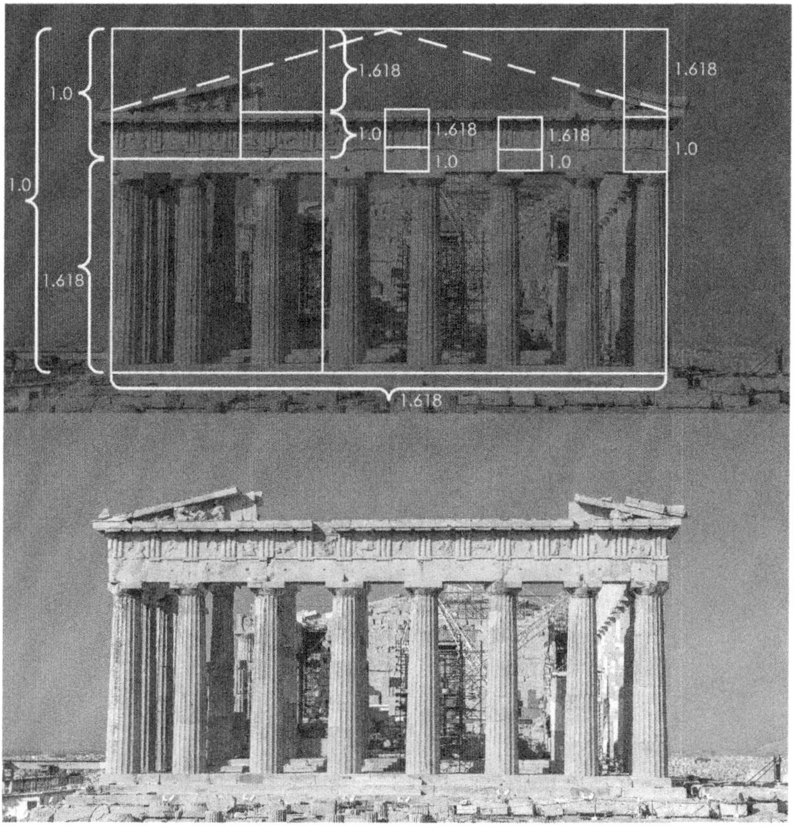

Figure 9. Parthenon (c. 432 BC) with (upper image) and without (lower image) golden ratio relationships within the architectural structure labeled.

Other ancient architectural structures thought to have golden ratio elements within their design include the Colosseum (Rome), Triumphal Arch of Constantine (Rome), Stonehenge (England), Pyramid of Niches (Mexico), Pyramid of the Sun (Mexico), El Castillo in Chichen Itza (Mexico), the Ziggurat of Babylon (Iraq), and the Ziggurat of Ur (Iraq).[4]

The Laon Cathedral in France is an early French Gothic cathedral whose construction began in the late 12th century. In the early 1900s, Frederik Lund published a detailed sketch of this cathedral (Figure 10) and argued that golden ratio relationships existed extensively within the Laon Cathedral's architecture.[5] Modern analysis of the architecture of the Laon Cathedral seems to agree with Lund's assertations (Figure 11).

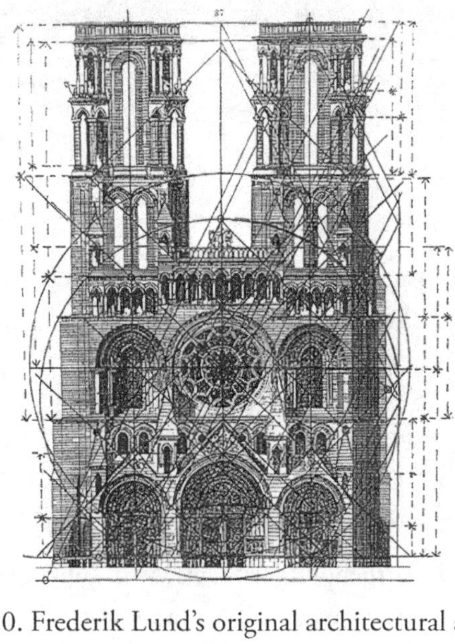

Figure 10. Frederik Lund's original architectural schematic of the Laon Cathedral. Golden ratio relationships are meticulously illustrated throughout the structure in this drawing.[5]

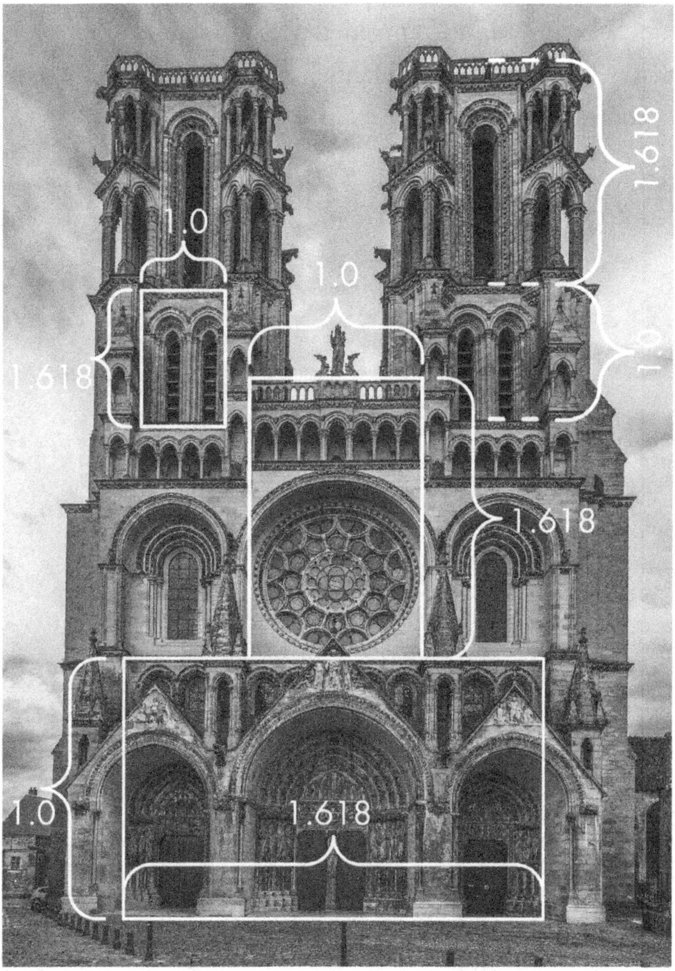

Figure 11. Laon Cathedral in Laon, France. Golden ratio relationships, including golden rectangles, are labeled with brackets and the numbers 1.618 and 1.0.

The Notre-Dame Cathedral in Paris, France, is another similar French Gothic cathedral whose construction began in the 12th century. The Notre-Dame Cathedral is the most famous of the

Gothic cathedrals and is considered a national symbol of France. Hidden within the Notre-Dame Cathedral are multiple golden ratio proportions (Figure 12).

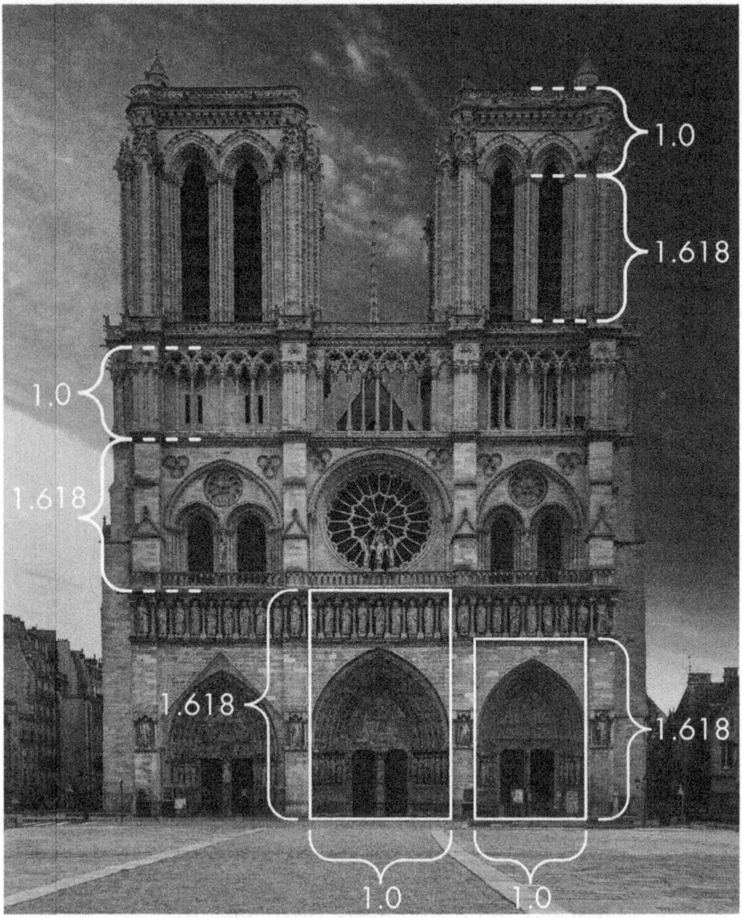

Figure 12. Notre-Dame Cathedral in Paris, France. Golden ratio proportions, including golden rectangles, are labeled with brackets and with the numbers 1.618 and 1.0 within the structure.[6]

Golden ratio relationships are also seen in modern architectural design. Le Corbusier, a French architect and city planner, created a complex measurement system called the "Modulor." This measurement system was essentially the combination of the metric decimal system and the foot-based Anglo-Saxon (imperial) system related to the anatomic proportions of a stylized human male figure. Golden ratio relationships within the human figure of the Modulor exist between the bottom of the foot, the navel, and the top of the head. Another golden ratio relationship exists between the navel, the top of the head, and the tip of the fingers in the outstretched left arm of the figure (Figure 13). Le Corbusier was involved in the design of the United Nations Secretariat Building in New York (Figure 14).

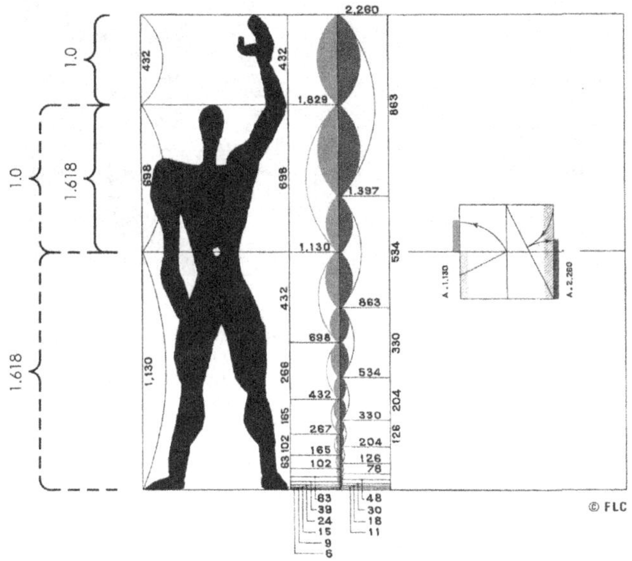

Figure 13. Modulor by Le Corbusier[7] (1945). Golden ratio proportion labeling added to the left side of the Modulor with brackets and the numbers 1.618 and 1.0. (Image used with permission, ©F.L.C./ADAGP, Paris/ Artists Rights Society (ARS), New York 2020)

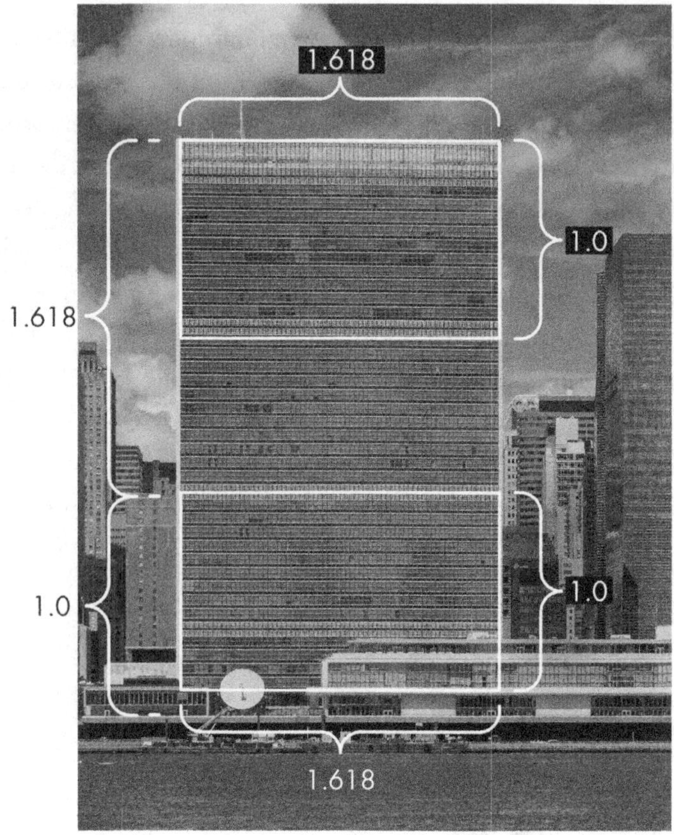

Figure 14. United Nations Secretariat Building in New York. Le Corbusier was involved in the design of this building. Hidden golden rectangles and a vertical golden ratio relationship are labeled within the structure with brackets and the numbers 1.618 and 1.0.

The Golden Ratio in Fine Art

Golden ratio relationships can be found in the composition of an astounding number of the world's most famous works of fine art. As previously mentioned in Chapter 1, Leonardo da Vinci famously illustrated the book written by mathematician Luca Pacioli titled *De Divina Proportione* ("On the Divine Proportion"). Clearly, da Vinci was very well aware of the existence of the golden ratio because of his illustrative work for mathematician Pacioli. The Museum of Science in Boston, Massachusetts, created a fascinating educational website about the life and work of Leonardo da Vinci.[8] On this museum's website is an "Activities" section that allows the viewer to individually overlay golden ratio-based geometrical shapes, one at a time, on top of several of da Vinci's most famous works of art. The premise is that da Vinci secretly incorporated hidden, golden ratio design elements within his artistic masterpieces. Unfortunately, there's no way of truly knowing if da Vinci used golden ratio relationships while composing his masterpieces—short of an actual direct admission from the artist himself. Such an admission, however, doesn't exist.

The figures that follow reveal several golden ratio relationships that exist within Leonardo da Vinci's paintings as depicted on the interactive website.

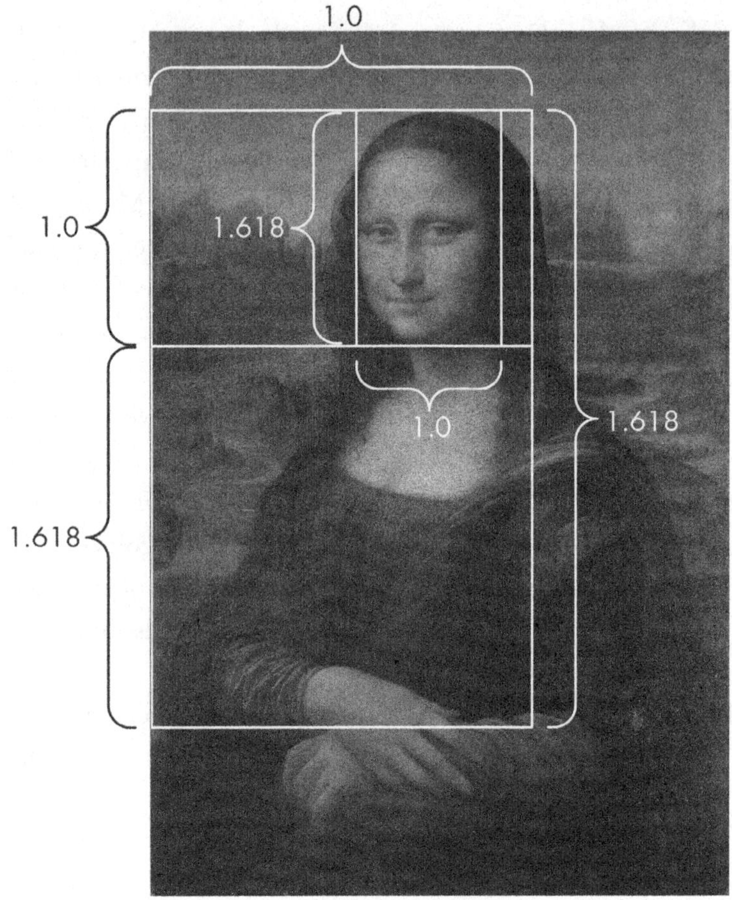

Figure 15. Mona Lisa by Leonardo da Vinci (c. 1503–1519). Golden ratio relationships within the work's composition are labeled with the numbers 1.618 and 1.0.

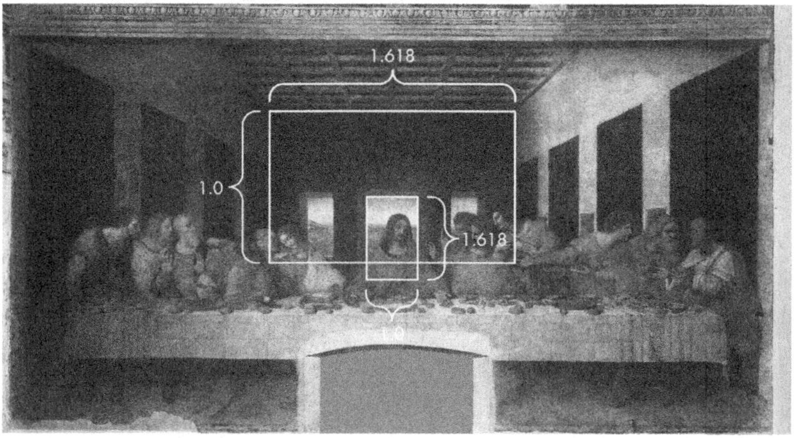

Figure 16. The Last Supper by Leonardo da Vinci (c. 1495–1498). Golden ratio relationships within the work's composition are labeled with the numbers 1.618 and 1.0.

Golden ratio relationships exist within the artwork of many other world-renowned artists. McGucken, a Princeton physicist and fine art photographer, described golden ratio relationships within the artwork of Michelangelo, Botticelli, Rembrandt, Picasso, Monet, Seurat, Dali, Rubens, and Vermeer.[9] Examples of some of these golden ratio relationships are depicted in the next group of figures.

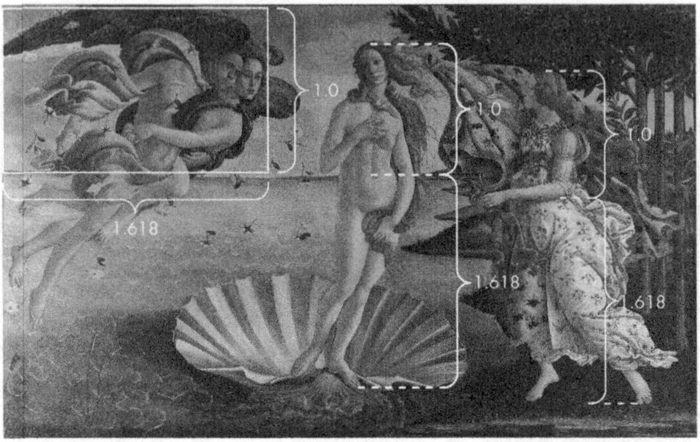

Figure 17. The Birth of Venus by Sandro Botticelli (c. 1485). Golden ratio relationships are labeled with the numbers 1.618 and 1.0.

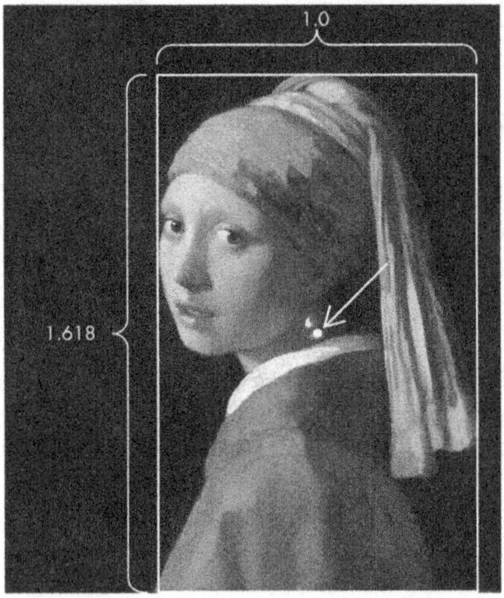

Figure 18. Girl with a Pearl Earring by Johanne Vermeer (c. 1665). The woman appears to be secretly framed within a golden rectangle. Her earring (arrow) is centered within this golden rectangle.[9]

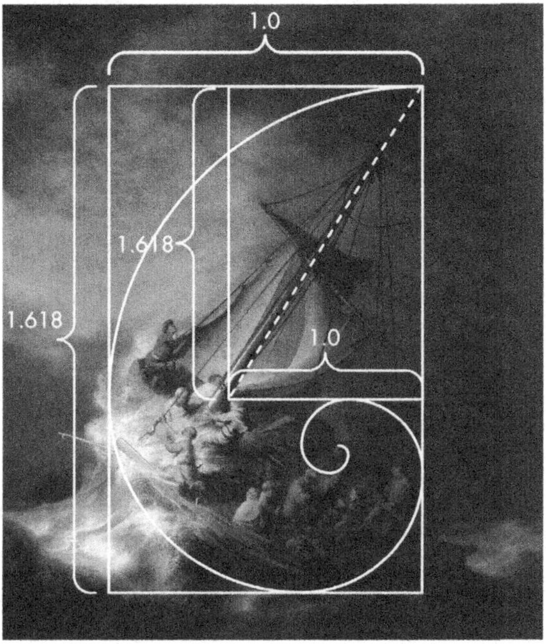

Figure 19. Christ in the Storm on the Sea of Galilee by Rembrandt van Rijn (1633). Several golden ratio relationships exist, including a diagonal (dashed line) within a golden rectangle that follows the tilt of the sailboat's mast. The golden spiral within the large, outer, golden rectangle appears to relate to the tilted position of the boat and the immediately adjacent clouds.[9]

The Mathematics of the Golden Ratio

The Greek mathematician, Euclid of Alexandria, is thought to be the first to formally describe the golden ratio. Euclid is often referred to as the "father of geometry." In his book *Elements* (c. 300 BC), Euclid is credited with the first attempt at a written definition of the golden ratio, which he described as an "extreme and mean ratio." Euclid wrote, "A straight line is said to have been cut in extreme and mean ratio when, as the whole line is to the greater segment, so is the greater to the less."[10]

As mentioned in Chapter 1, the Greek letter phi (either upper case ϕ or lower case φ) is the most common symbol used today to symbolize the golden ratio. Phi has been used to symbolize the golden ratio ever since the early 1900s.[11] In academic mathematical literature, the Greek letter tau (τ), meaning "the section," is also commonly used to symbolize the golden ratio.

Two numbers can form a golden ratio if their ratio equals the ratio of their sum to the larger of the two numbers. In the equations below, *a* and *b* represent two numbers that can form the golden ratio, and *a* is larger than *b*. Therefore, the golden ratio is as follows:

$$\frac{a+b}{a} = \frac{a}{b} = \phi$$

The golden ratio takes on a specific numerical value,

$$\phi = \frac{1.618}{1} = 1.618$$

or, expressed as is common for a ratio, 1.618…:1 = 1.618…

To better understand the golden ratio, I believe it's helpful to look at the golden ratio relationship linearly. The golden ratio relationship exists if we divide a line segment into two unequal sub-lengths. The longer section (a) of the line divided by the shorter section (b) of the line is equal to the total line length (a+b) divided by the longer section (a). This is referred to as the golden section (Figure 20).

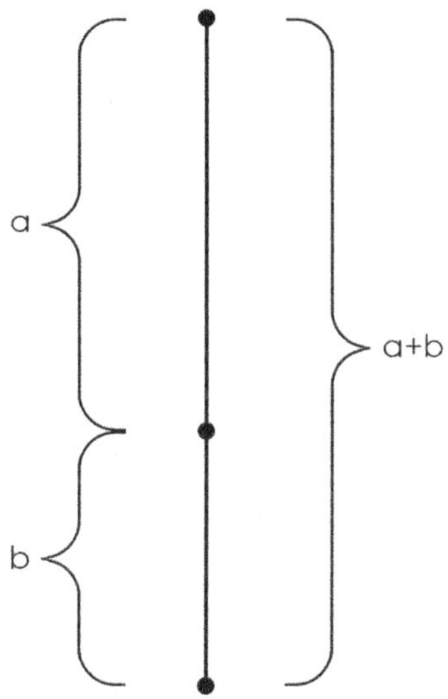

Figure 20. Golden section.

If the shorter section (b) were assumed to have a length of 1.0, then, for the two line segments to have a golden ratio relationship, the longer segment (a) would have a length of 1.618. The ratio of the two line segments would be 1.618:1.0, the golden section (Figure 21).

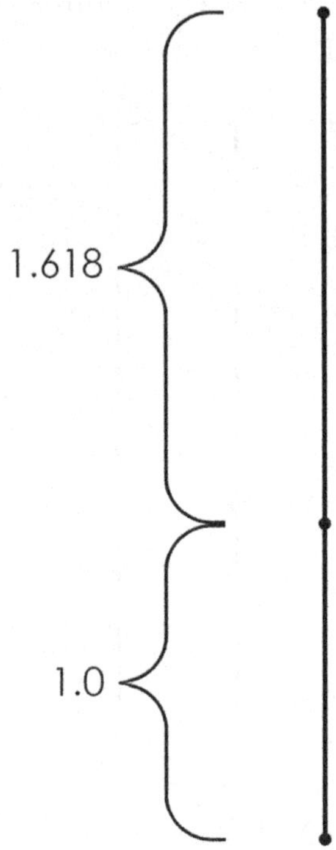

Figure 21. Golden section labeled with 1.618:1.0.

The golden ratio is an irrational number that's approximately equal to 1.618. In reality, this irrational number never ends (its decimal place keeps going on forever) and never repeats. Here, ϕ is shown with only eight of its infinite number of digits past the decimal: 1.61803399… For ease of use, ϕ is typically shown as the rounded, and therefore approximate, value of 1.618. I use this rounded value throughout this treatise.

The Golden Rectangle

The golden rectangle is a rectangle in which the ratio of the long side's length to that of the short side reduces to 1.618/1.0 = 1.618:1.0 (i.e., long side:short side). This is illustrated in Figure 22.

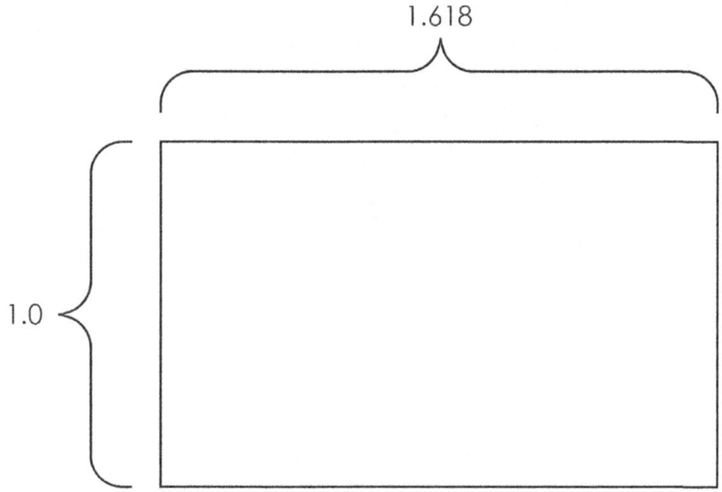

Figure 22. Golden rectangle.

A fascinating property of a golden rectangle is that, if a perfect square is removed from a golden rectangle, another golden rectangle is formed (Figure 23).

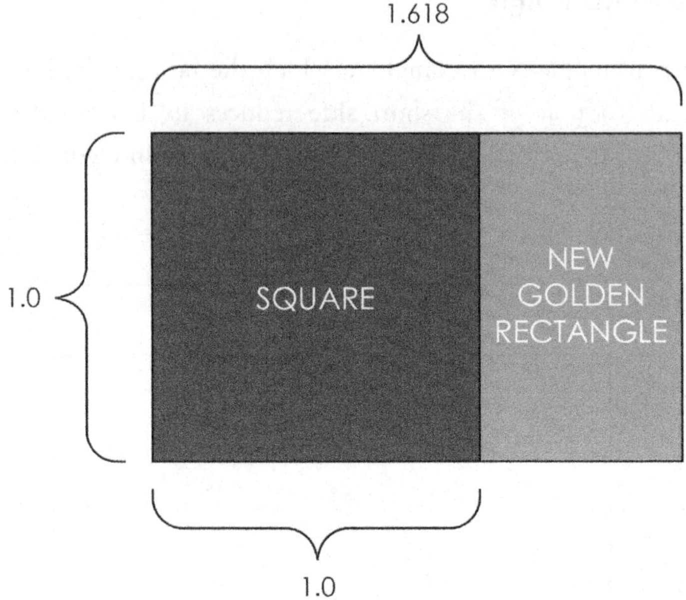

Figure 23. Large golden rectangle divided into a perfect square (dark gray) and a smaller golden rectangle (light gray).

In the series of images in Figure 24, imagine that we've successively removed a perfect square (dark gray) from the larger golden rectangle. By doing so, we create another golden rectangle (light gray), albeit smaller in size. The process of removing a perfect square from a smaller golden rectangle can continue indefinitely. Many progressively smaller golden rectangles can exist within the largest golden rectangle.

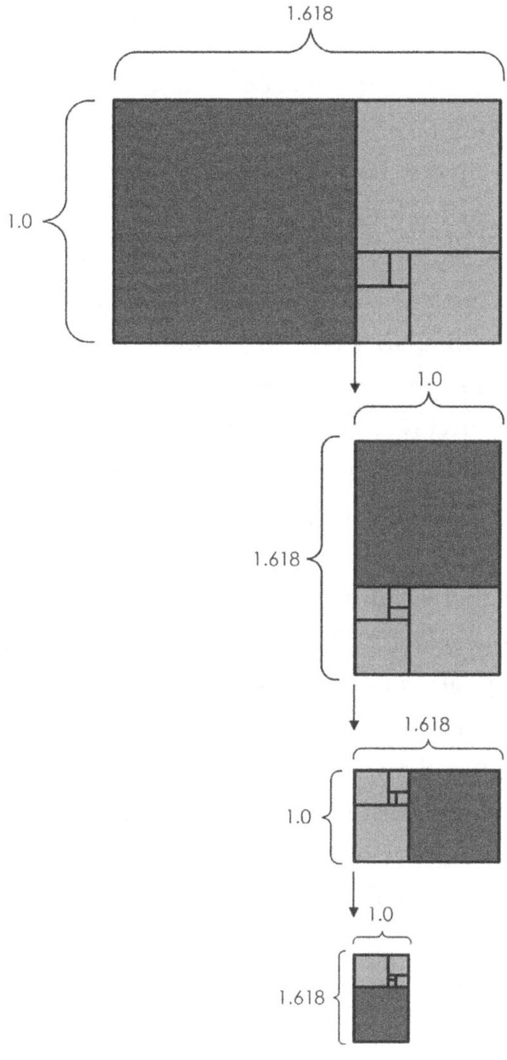

Figure 24. Series of golden rectangles created by the sequential removal of a perfect square from a golden rectangle. Although the lengths of the sides of the golden rectangles decrease as squares are sequentially removed, the ratio of the length of the long side to that of the short side in each of the smaller rectangles is a golden one.

The Logarithmic Spiral

Within these multiple, internal golden rectangles just described in Figure 24, a special type of spiral called a *logarithmic spiral* can be constructed. The famous 16th-century mathematician Jacob Bernoulli referred to the logarithmic spiral as *spira mirabilis*, the "marvelous spiral."[12]

Logarithmic spirals possess an interesting mathematical property known as self-similarity. The logarithmic spiral increases in size from its origin in geometric progression, but its shape doesn't change with each successive curve of the spiral. This process is like the one demonstrated in Figure 24, in which the rectangles were reduced by perfect squares to produce golden rectangles, only in reverse.

The golden spiral is a unique type of logarithmic spiral, as its growth factor is the golden ratio. As it forms a series of progressively larger golden spirals, for every quarter or 90° turn, the distance from the edge to the center of the spiral increases by the golden ratio $\phi = 1.618$, but the spiral retains its shape throughout this process. Thus, as the golden spiral becomes larger, its edge moves farther from its center, or origin, by a factor of 1.618 for every quarter turn that it grows. The golden spiral in Figure 25 originated from the corner of the square within the smallest golden rectangle.

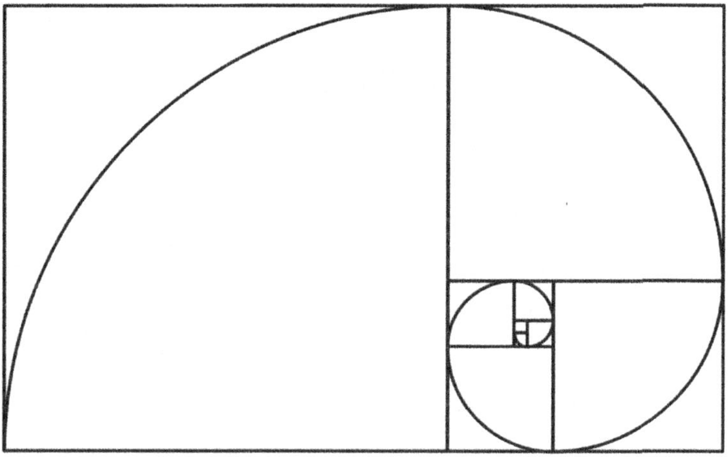

Figure 25. The golden spiral within a golden rectangle.

For the mathematically inclined, let's look a little closer at the growth of a golden spiral. In Figure 26, the golden spiral is shown on a Cartesian coordinate system centered on the point (0, 0). The coordinate system is divided into four areas by its two axes. The spiral begins its growth, which is centered at point (0, 0), at point (1, 0), and the movement of its growth is counterclockwise. To complete a quarter or 90° turn around the center of the coordinate system (0, 0), the spiral grows from its starting point of (1, 0) to point (0, 1.618) on the coordinate scale.

A rectangle, shown in gray, is plotted to represent this growth. We can use this rectangle to determine if the factor of the spiral's growth is indeed the golden ratio. The rectangle is formed by the points (0, 0), (1, 0), (1, 1.618), and (0, 1.618). As we can see, the ratio of the rectangle's long side to its short side, 1.618:1.0, forms the golden ratio.

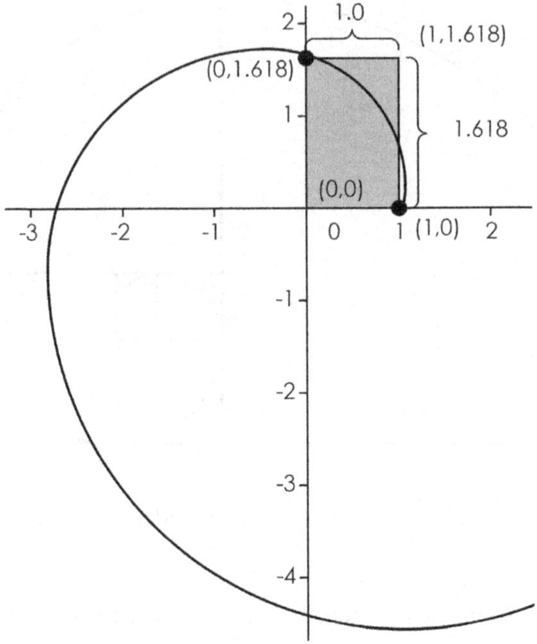

Figure 26. Growth of the golden spiral: first quarter turn.

Figure 27 shows the spiral's growth from point (0, 1.618) to point (-2.618, 0) on the coordinate scale, representing another counterclockwise quarter turn around its origin of (0, 0). Again, I've included a rectangle, shown in darker gray to plot this growth. From right to left, the points defining this rectangle are (0, 0), (0,1.618), (-2.618, 1.618), and (-2.618, 0). Notice that the spiral maintains its spiral shape as it grows.

Does the golden ratio represent the growth of the spiral from (0, 1.618) to (-2.618, 0)? Let's use the rectangle we've plotted to find out.

As shown in Figure 27, the rectangle's sides have lengths of

2.618 and 1.618, and so the ratio of these lengths with the higher length first and the shorter last is 2.618:1.618. Dividing this yields 1.618 when rounded, or the close approximation of the golden mean commonly adopted. These numbers also satisfy the part of the golden ratio's definition that says:

$$\frac{a + b}{a}$$

$$\frac{2.618 + 1.618}{2.618} = 1.618 \ldots$$

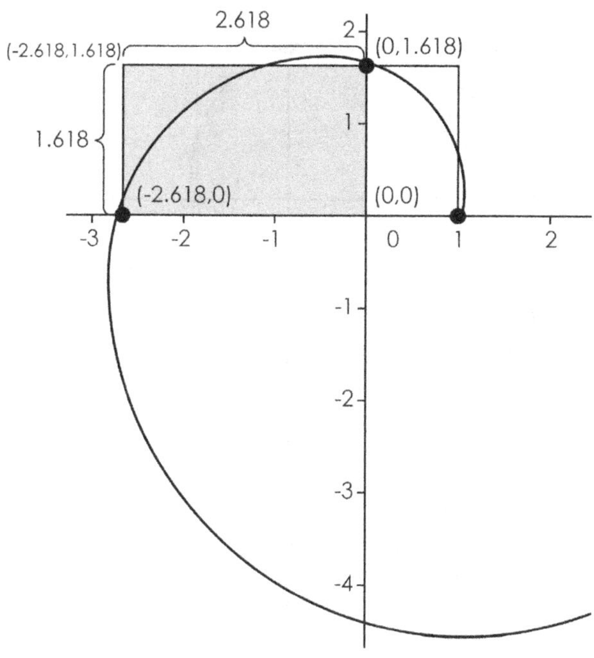

Figure 27. Growth of the golden spiral: second quarter turn.

Let's look at one more counterclockwise quarter turn of the spiral's growth (Figure 28). This time, its growth takes it from point (-2.618, 0) to point (0, -4.236). I again plot a rectangle to match the spiral's growth. Its points, from right to left, are at (0, 0), (-2.618, 0), (-2.618, -4.236), and (0, -4.236). This is illustrated in Figure 28 below.

Let's see if the ratio of the rectangle's sides, and hence the growth of the spiral from (-2.618, 0) to (0, -4.236), is according to the golden ratio. We make a ratio of the rectangle's sides, long side first, 4.236:2.618, and divide. The result is 1.618..., an irrational number close enough to the golden ratio to be shown as the ratio's typical estimate of 1.618.

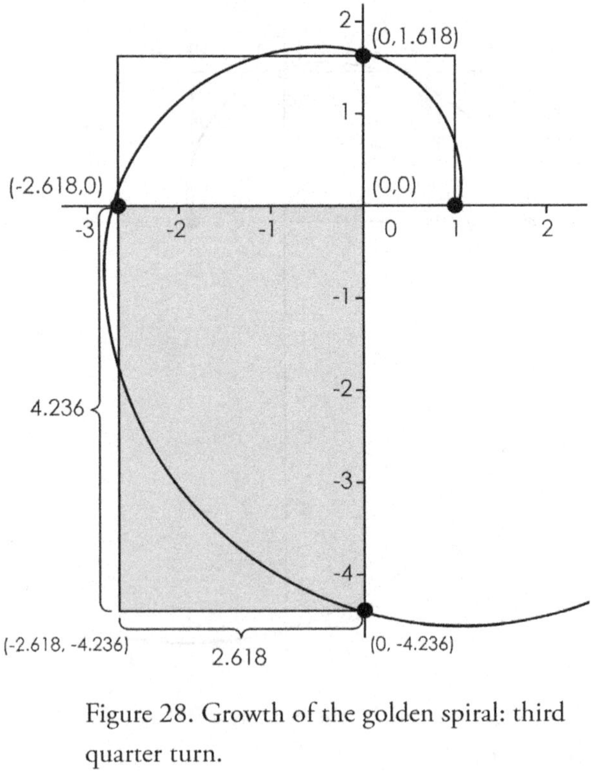

Figure 28. Growth of the golden spiral: third quarter turn.

Again, let's verify these numbers using the other part of the golden ratio's mathematical definition:

$$\frac{a + b}{a}$$

$$\frac{4.236 + 2.618}{4.236} = 1.618 \ldots$$

The spiral would continue to grow until interrupted, retaining its spiral shape and increasing the distance from the origin (0, 0) to the spiral's edge at each quarter turn by 1.618 from the previous quarter turn's distance.

The Golden Ratio in Nature

Surprisingly, logarithmic spirals actually exist in nature. Patterns in nature can be thought of as consistencies of form that repeat themselves in the natural world. The examples I've given thus far of golden ratio relationships are within man-made, artificial creations in which humans were in full control of creating the dimensions of the object (e.g., graphic arts, paintings, and architecture). Logarithmic spiral patterns, however, abound in nature. Examples include nautilus shells, swirls of hurricanes, spiral galaxies, and even plants (Figure 29).

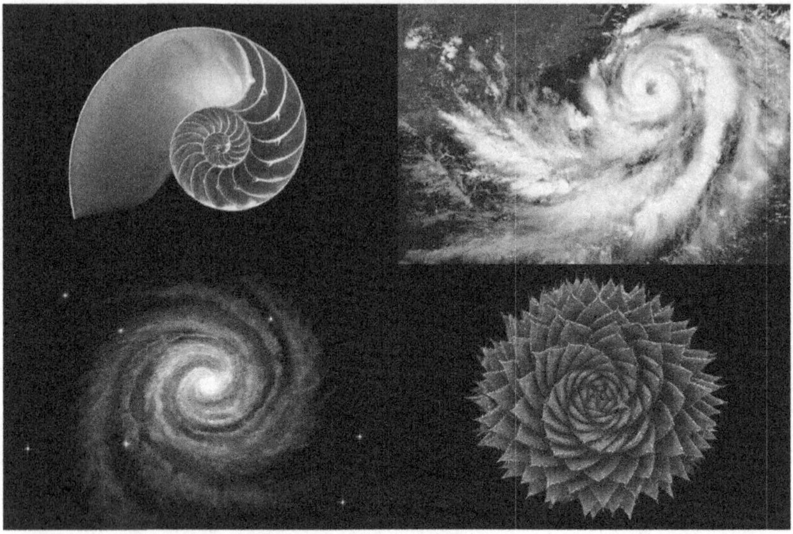

Figure 29. Examples of logarithmic spirals in nature. Nautilus shell (upper left), hurricane (upper right), Milky Way galaxy (lower left), and an aloe vera plant (lower right).

Fibonacci numbers, also called the *Fibonacci sequence*, are a sequence of numbers in which each number in the sequence is the sum of the previous two numbers. The Fibonacci sequence, starting from 0, is 0, 1, 1, 2, 3, 5, 8, 13, 21, 34, 55, etc. The ratio of successive pairs of numbers in this sequence progressively approaches 1.618. The higher we go in the Fibonacci sequence, the closer we get to a ratio of two successive numbers that yield 1.618. For example, the ratio of 5/3 (a pair of successive low numbers early in the Fibonacci sequence) is 1.666... If we go higher in the Fibonacci sequence, the ratio of the pair of successive numbers 55/34 is 1.617... Even higher in the Fibonacci sequence, the ratio of the pair of successive numbers 233/144 is 1.618...

The golden ratio and the closely related Fibonacci sequence can be found in flower petal growth patterns, the seed heads of sunflowers, pinecones, pineapples, cauliflower, tree branch growth patterns, and even the DNA molecule. Proportional analysis of fish, Dungeness crabs, clams, stingrays, beetles, butterflies, frog skeletons, horse skeletons, and even dinosaur skeletons all show golden ratio elements.[4] Most importantly, the golden ratio also seems to exist within attractive human anatomy. As we'll explore later in this treatise, I believe that the golden ratio exists extensively within the anatomic features of beautiful human faces and breasts.

CHAPTER 3

DIVINE FACE®

Beauty Analysis of the Human Face Based on the Golden Ratio

I have created a patented system and method that analyzes the physical appearance of the human face.[1,2] My facial analysis methodology is based on golden ratio relationships hidden within specific sets of facial anatomic features. Hayduke Facial Grids are a set of digital grids that are overlaid on facial images of the client being tested. These overlay grids are used as the core mechanism of my facial analysis methodology.

Hayduke Facial Grid designs are based on specific sets of golden ratio facial anatomic relationships as well as right and left sided symmetry of human facial anatomic features. If the measured distances between the anatomic features of the client's image align with the specific requirements of the Hayduke Facial Grid being tested, the client scores a "successful" fit for that particular Hayduke Facial Grid. If the client's facial anatomic features don't meet the strict location requirements of the Hayduke Facial Grid being tested, the client fails that particular Hayduke Facial Grid.

Hayduke Facial Grids form the foundation of the Hayduke Facial Analysis test of beauty and physical attractiveness. The

Hayduke Facial Analysis test generates a score that reflects how many golden ratio relationships exist within a client's facial features based on extensive testing with a battery of patented Hayduke Facial Grids. Facial symmetry between right- and left-sided facial anatomic features is also reflected in the results of a Hayduke Facial Analysis. The Hayduke Facial Analysis test can be easily applied to human digital facial images via application software that I created called Divine Face®.

Image Capture Guidelines

The first step in my facial analysis methodology requires capturing high-resolution digital images of the client's face. Digital images of the client's face from three specific poses (frontal, right profile, and left profile) are then uploaded into the Divine Face® application software. The most common type of digital images currently used in my personal plastic surgery practice are high-resolution, two-dimensional, digital still photographs. Three-dimensional digital photographs and digital video images are other types of digital images that can also be applied to my methodology. As image-capture technology advances, the quality and resolution of facial digital images will also improve. The Hayduke Facial Analysis will continue to be applicable to any future image-capture technological advances. In fact, future technological improvements in image clarity will surely improve visualization of finer anatomic details within the facial digital images. This improved anatomic detail will also serve to improve the overall accuracy of the Hayduke Facial Analysis.

Proper facial image capture guidelines require that the client's hair be pulled back behind the ears and completely away from their face. The client's forehead, natural hairline, and ears should be fully exposed. This usually requires a ponytail hairstyle for women with long hair. Men with long hair may be required to slick their hair back with either water or a strong gel-type hair product to completely expose their hairline and ears. Jewelry should be totally absent from the images. Clients aren't allowed to wear makeup or eyelash extensions. Images should be framed from just above the top of the head to just below the level of the clavicles, with the neck fully exposed. Ideally, clothing should be absent from the image, including any type of clothing that obscures the clavicles and neck. The best results are obtained if the client's shirt is removed before capturing the facial images.

Facial images (photographs, videos, etc.) used within the Divine Face® application software currently require frontal, right profile, and left profile poses. The facial expression of the client should be totally neutral. The client shouldn't be smiling or frowning when the images are captured. The client's lips should be gently closed and the teeth should be in full occlusion. Each image should ideally include a calibrated metric ruler within the image on the same plane as the client's face. The ruler shouldn't obscure any part of the face or neck. The client can be simply asked to hold a ruler near their face at the time of image capture.

Digital single-lens reflex (DSLR) or digital mirrorless cameras, both with interchangeable lens capability, are currently recommended for capturing high-resolution two-dimensional digital facial images. To minimize image distortion, the facial digital image capture properties should be equivalent to photographs taken with a 90 to 105 mm focal length lens on a single lens reflex 35 mm film camera. This guideline is considered an accepted standard for clinical plastic surgery facial photography.[3] The crop factor of the specific digital camera's image sensor must be known in order to choose the proper digital camera lens focal length to achieve this goal. Using the wrong lens focus length to capture the facial images distorts the client's anatomy within the images. This will lead to less accurate test results.

The ideal lighting for capturing facial images is "flat lighting" that doesn't create any significant dark shadows on the client's face or neck. Studio lighting with multiple lights is preferred to achieve flat lighting. For single light source situations, the camera's flash should not be pointed directly at the client's face but rather bounced off of the ceiling to help flatten the lighting. Strong shadows on the face and neck obscure anatomic detail that is required for a quality facial analysis. If the facial image has too much shadowing and contrast, some of the finer anatomic details will be lost within the dark shadows. White balancing should be performed to capture the most realistic colors if color images are taken. If the camera's automatic white balance feature is accurate, that will suffice. The camera lens should be kept directly level with the client's face when capturing the facial image. Ideally, a tripod should be used to avoid camera movement during image capture. The resolution of the images should be as high as the digital camera and technology allow.

Basic client intake information as well as specific measurements obtained directly from the client's physical examination are manually entered into the client database section of the Divine Face® application software. Scanned or photographed documents—such as signed consent forms, model-image releases, and copies of identification cards—may also be uploaded into the database section.

Labeling Facial Images with Anatomic Markers

The next step in the analysis involves accurate placement of overlay anatomic markers (digital dots) on specific anatomic facial landmarks of the captured digital images. The facial digital images have several automatic anatomic landmarks that are immediately superimposed upon the uploaded images via computer vision technology. For example, anatomic landmark markers on the pupils are automatically generated on those specific anatomic structures of the captured facial images without assistance from the application software user. In addition to these automatically generated facial anatomic landmark markers, several other anatomic landmark markers must be manually positioned by the Divine Face® user. The application software user uses a reference image with properly placed anatomic markers (digital dots) to guide the manual landmark positioning process on the images being tested. This reference image for each pose is located on the left side of the computer screen, while the client's uploaded image is located on the right side of the computer screen. Each facial landmark overlay marker must be fine-tuned by the user and repositioned into the final proper resting position. The final, approved, resting position of the landmark overlay marker must be formally confirmed by the user in order to proceed. Once the landmark overlay marker position is formally approved by the user, the digital dots change color from red to green.

The measurement scale is then set using the "set scale" tool within the Divine Face® application software. The measurement scale is the reference scale that allows the Divine Face® application to measure accurate distances within the captured images. Measurement scale setting can be achieved by using either the image of the metric ruler (that was included within each original facial image) or via specific anatomic measurements derived from direct physical examination of the client's face. After achieving proper scale-setting confirmation for all three poses of the facial digital images, the client's face can now be tested with a battery of Hayduke Facial Grids.

Analyzing Facial Images with Hayduke Facial Grids

For facial analysis, multiple Hayduke Facial Grids are used to analyze the facial digital images of the client. At this point, all the anatomic landmarks on the images being tested have been marked with overlay markers (digital dots), and the measurement scale has been set. Each Hayduke Facial Grid is based upon the relationship of the golden ratio within the grid to a specific set of defined facial anatomic landmarks that have already been marked with digital dots on the client's digital images. Each individual Hayduke Facial Grid in my series is composed of a unique set of anatomic landmarks and assigned a unique identifying grid number.

An example of a simple grid within my facial grid series is Hayduke Facial Grid 15 (Figure 30). This grid consists of two vertically arranged quadrilaterals (rectangles) derived from three horizontal gridlines. The horizontal gridline positions are determined by a specific set of anatomic landmarks that are labeled with overlay markers (digital dots) on a frontal image of the client. The anatomic landmarks that define Hayduke Facial Grid 15 include anatomic landmarks at the eyebrow arch peaks (labeled as 319 in Figure 30), the upper eyelid margin (labeled as 318 in Figure 30), and the lower eyelid margin (labeled as 317 in Figure 30). Based on these specific anatomic landmarks, Hayduke Facial Grid 15 is overlaid on the client's digital image.

The relation of the lengths of the vertical sides of the two quadrilaterals within Hayduke Facial Grid 15 determines the success or failure of the fit of this grid. After the grid is overlaid onto the client's frontal digital image, the lengths of the two vertical sides of the vertically arranged quadrilaterals of Hayduke Facial Grid 15 are automatically measured by the application software.

The vertical distances between the three horizontal gridlines of the client being tested are measured first in millimeters and then reduced to a ratio. In order for a client's face to be scored as a "successful" fit of Hayduke Facial Grid 15, the client's anatomical structures would need to be related to each other in such a way that the vertical distances between the horizontal gridlines would reduce to a ratio of 1.0:1.618. In the schematic of Hayduke Facial Grid 15 (Figure 30), the lowermost quadrilateral's vertical side is labeled 1.0. The uppermost quadrilateral's vertical side is labeled with 1.618. These numbers, 1.0 and 1.618, reflect what the ratio of the lengths of these two sides should be in an ideal "successful" fit of Hayduke Facial Grid 15.

If the client being tested has, for example, very low eyebrows (or eyebrows that are too high on the forehead), then the ratio of the vertical side measurements wouldn't equal 1.0:1.618. In that situation, the grid would be scored as a "failed" grid. With low eyebrows, for example, the vertical side of the upper quadrilateral may have a value of 1.274 and thus result in a failure of fit for Hayduke Facial Grid 15.

A successful fit of Hayduke Facial Grid 15 is depicted in Figure 31. The professional model in Figure 31 has anatomic features, specified in Hayduke Facial Grid 15, that are indeed related to each other by a ratio of 1.0:1.618. In her case, Hayduke Facial Grid 15 would be scored as a "successful" fit, and she would receive one point toward the total score of a Hayduke Facial Analysis.

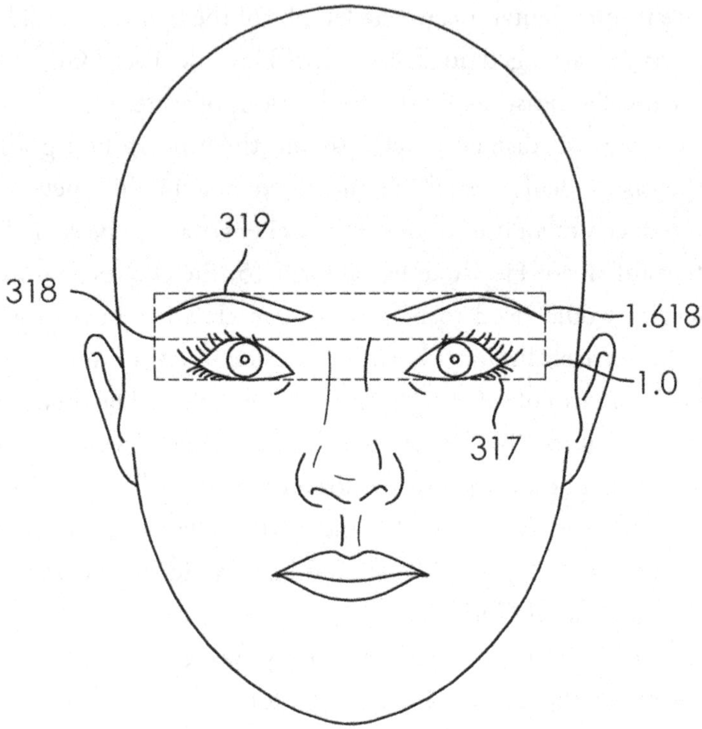

Figure 30. Hayduke Facial Grid 15.

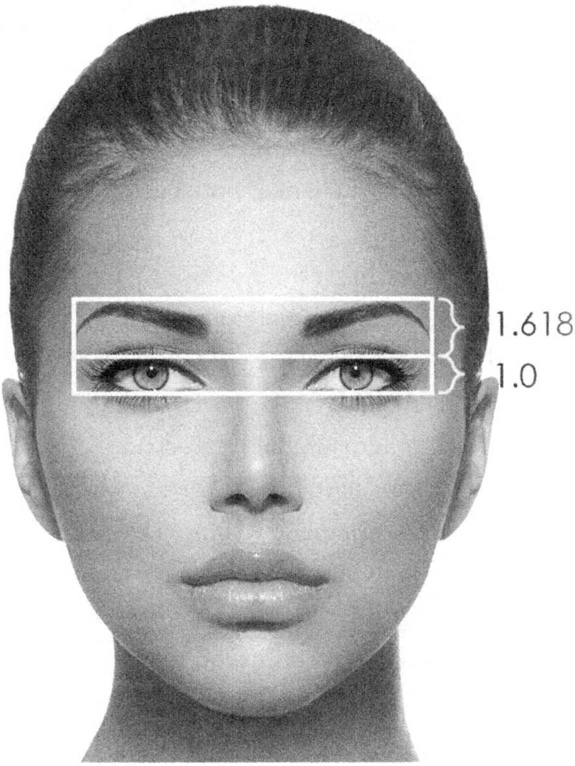

Figure 31. Professional model with a successful fit for Hayduke Facial Grid 15.

Another example of a simple grid within my facial grid series is Hayduke Facial Grid 11 (Figure 32). This grid also consists of two vertically arranged quadrilaterals derived from three horizontal gridlines. The anatomic landmarks within the schematic that define the gridline location of Hayduke Facial Grid 11 include anatomic landmarks at the peaks of the eyebrow arches (labeled as 307 in Figure 32), the upper lip vermillion apex plane (labeled as 301 in Figure 32), and the inferior margin of the chin (labeled as 306 in Figure 32). These anchor points guide the placement of the three horizontal gridlines of Hayduke Facial Grid 11. For a successful fit of this grid, the lengths of the vertical sides of the two vertically arranged quadrilaterals should be related by the ratio 1.0:1.618, as depicted in the grid's schematic (Figure 32).

The professional female model in Figure 33 has anatomic features, based on the specific set of previously defined anatomic landmarks, that fit the golden ratio requirements of Hayduke Facial Grid 11. Hayduke Facial Grid 11 would be scored as a "successful" fit for this professional model. She would receive one point toward the total score of a Hayduke Facial Analysis for a successful fit of Hayduke Facial Grid 11.

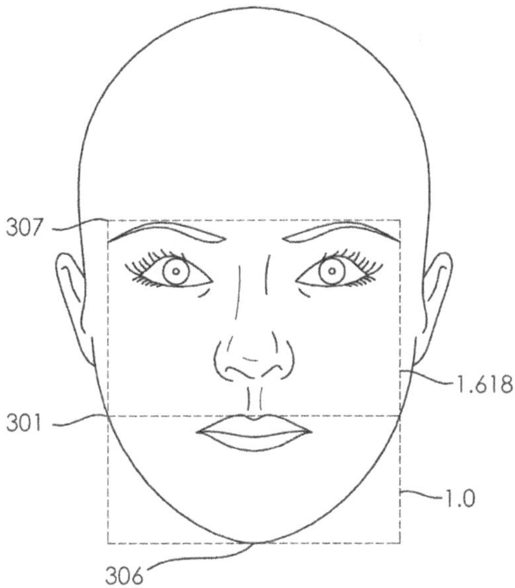

Figure 32. Hayduke Facial Grid 11.

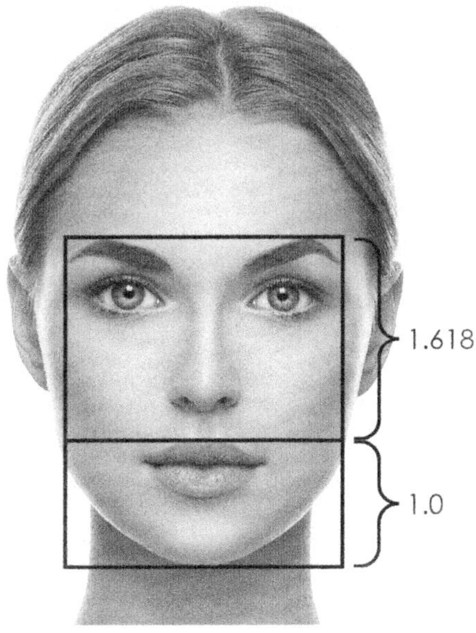

Figure 33. Professional model with a successful fit for Hayduke Facial Grid 11.

Hayduke Facial Grid 4 (Figure 34) is another example of a simple grid in my series. The three horizontal gridlines of this grid are defined in the schematic by the nasal base plane (labeled as 313 in Figure 34), the upper lip vermillion apex plane (labeled as 301 in Figure 34), and the inferior margin of the lower lip (labeled as 303 in Figure 34). A successful fit of this grid is shown in the professional female model depicted in Figure 35. She would receive one point toward the total score of a Hayduke Facial Analysis for a successful fit of Hayduke Facial Grid 4.

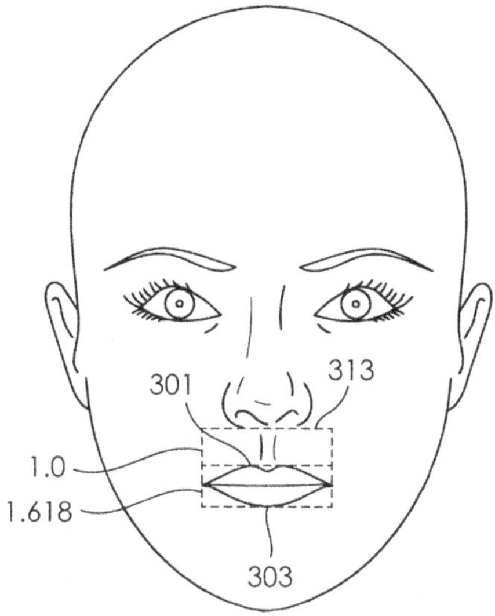

Figure 34. Hayduke Facial Grid 4.

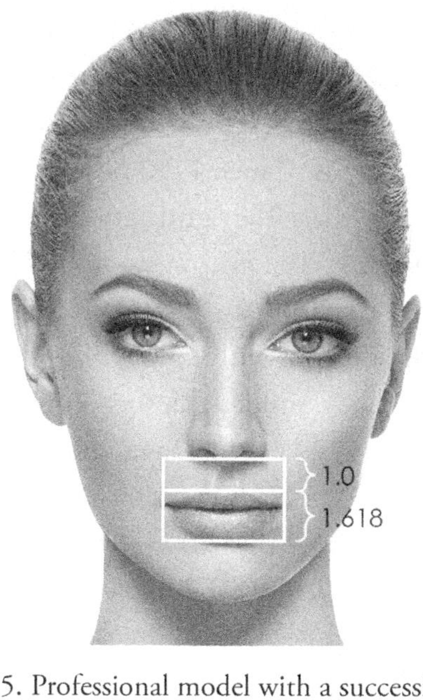

Figure 35. Professional model with a successful fit for Hayduke Facial Grid 4.

Generating a Hayduke Facial Analysis Test Score Report

After choosing which specific Hayduke Facial Grids to test, a Hayduke Facial Analysis test score report may be requested by the Divine Face® user. The Hayduke Facial Analysis test score report displays the names of the successful grids and failed grids from the specific grids chosen for testing. These results are displayed as three "section" scores (frontal, right profile, and left profile) as well as a "total" score for all three sections combined. The total Hayduke Facial Analysis test score is displayed as a percentage of successful grids as well as a numerical fraction of successful grids to total grids tested. In addition, the percentage of successful grids and the ratios of successful grids to failed grids are displayed individually for each of the three sections (frontal, right profile, and left profile).

For each section, the specific grid names of the successful grids and failed grids are displayed as well as the "degree of grid fit" of each grid. The degree of grid fit, reported in parentheses after the specific successful grid name, reports how close a successful grid is to an absolutely perfect fit (range 1–1000, with 1000 reflecting an absolutely perfect grid fit). The "grid ratio offset" setting can also be adjusted by the user. The grid ratio offset setting reflects how much the grids can vary from an absolutely perfect fit of the specified 1.0:1.618 relationships within the grids tested (expressed as a percentage) and still be considered a successful grid fit. The other setting that can be adjusted by the Divine Face® user is the "grid rotational offset setting." The grid rotational offset setting dictates the specific degree of rotational tilt within a grid that's allowed for the grid to be scored as successful. This allows for some unintentional tilt (rotation) in the client's image at the time of image capture.

At the end of the session, a Divine Face® Hayduke Facial Analysis test "score report" can be printed out. The printed hard copy can be given to the client or saved in the patient's physical file (chart). This score report includes identifying information such as the client's name, image (photograph) date, date of birth, client's age at the time of image capture, height, and weight. The client's data are also stored automatically at the end of the test within the Divine Face® application software. Saved data include the confirmed anatomic landmark positions on all of the client's uploaded digital images.

Additions and revisions to the design of individual Hayduke Facial Grids and to the Divine Face® application software are constantly being implemented to achieve maximal analytic quality of the Hayduke Facial Analysis test.

(Detailed technical descriptions of each individual Hayduke Facial Grid are presented in the section below. Some readers may choose to skip this technical section and proceed to the next chapter.)

Technical Specifications of Individual Hayduke Facial Grids

Hayduke Facial Grids and the specific combination of anatomic landmarks involved in each grid's design are the core elements of my patented system and method of analyzing human facial anatomy (US Patent Nos. 9,721,146 and 9,996,943). Hayduke Facial Grid designs involved in the current version of the Hayduke Facial Analysis are detailed below. The facial schematics illustrate a simplified general anatomic layout of the individual golden ratio facial grids; however, the schematics do not actually harbor the 1.618:1.0 ratio within the illustrations' drawn dimensions. Written descriptions of the anatomic landmarks involved in each specific gridline are also defined to correspond to the numerical labels within the schematics of each Hayduke Facial Grid. Each grid schematic also has labels that include the numbers 1.618 and 1.0 to correspond to the required location of the golden ratio within the components of the grid. The location of the 1.618:1.0 ratio within a grid varies depending on the design of the grid. Some of the grids have the 1.618:1.0 ratio in the vertical components of the grid, and some grids harbor this ratio in the horizontal components. Several of the grids are combination grids that manifest the 1.618:1.0 relationship in both the vertical and horizontal components. Table 1 lists the anatomic descriptions that correspond to the reference numbers used in the Hayduke Facial Grid schematics.

Reference Number	Anatomic Description
301	upper lip vermillion apex plane at the Cupid's bow peaks
302	separation point of the lips
303	inferior margin of the lower lip vermillion apex plane
305	pupillary horizontal plane
306	inferior margin of the chin
307	peak of the eyebrow arch
308	left pupil
309	right pupil
310	medial canthus
311	contralateral medial canthus
312	medial canthal plane
313	nasal base plane
314	supratip breakpoint of the nose
316	center of the nostril opening
317	lower eyelid margin
318	upper eyelid margin
319	peak of the eyebrow arch
320	outer margin of the temporal process of the zygoma
321	contralateral temporal process of the zygoma
322	facial midline
323	contralateral lateral canthus
324	medial ipsilateral iris margin
325	ipsilateral medial canthus
326	right oral commissure
327	right Cupid's bow peak
328	left Cupid's bow peak
329	left oral commissure
330	ipsilateral lateral canthus
331	lateral ipsilateral iris margin
332	lateral canthus
333	nasal radix
334	anterior margin of the nasal tip
336	base of the upper lip philtral dimple
337	anterior margin of the eyeball
338	nose supratip break point
339	anterior margin of the chin
342	horizontal plane just above the nostril openings
346	inner margin of the nostril opening

Table 1. Anatomic descriptions corresponding to the reference numbers used in the Hayduke Facial Grid schematics.

Hayduke Facial Grid 1 (Figure 36) has three anchor points (anatomic landmarks) that dictate the location of the three horizontal gridlines of this grid. The first anchor point is located on the upper lip vermillion apex plane at the Cupid's bow peaks (301). This point dictates the location of the uppermost horizontal gridline. The second anchor point is located at the separation point of the lips (302). This point dictates the location of the middle horizontal gridline. The third anchor point is located on the lower lip vermillion apex plane (303). This point dictates the location of the lowermost horizontal gridline. The grid derived from these three anchor points consists of two vertically arranged quadrilaterals. The first quadrilateral is formed between the upper lip vermillion apex plane (301) and the separation point of the lips (302). The second quadrilateral is formed between the separation point of the lips (302) and the lower lip vermillion apex plane (303). The vertical side of the first quadrilateral is related to the vertical side of the second quadrilateral by the ratio 1.0:1.618.

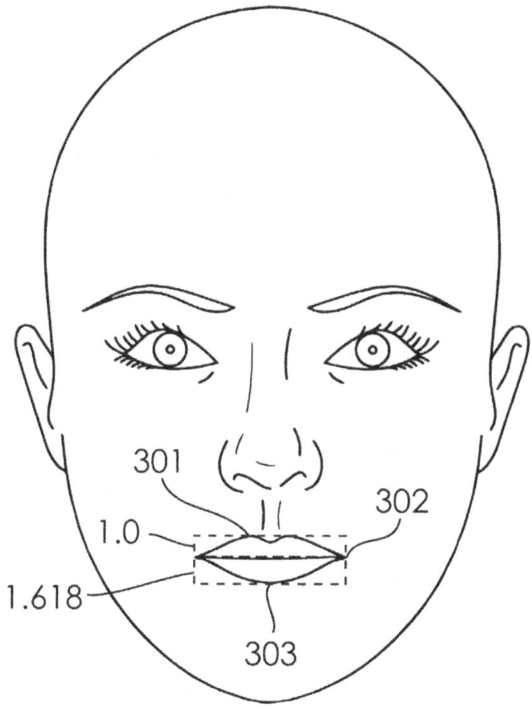

Figure 36. Hayduke Facial Grid 1.

Hayduke Facial Grid 2 (Figure 37) is composed of both horizontally and vertically arranged quadrilaterals. Three anchor points (anatomic landmarks) dictate the location of the horizontal gridlines of this grid. The first anchor point is located on the upper lip vermillion apex plane at the Cupid's bows peaks (301). The second anchor point is located at the separation point of the lips (302). The third anchor point is located on the lower lip vermillion apex plane (303). These three anchor points guide the formation of two vertically arranged quadrilaterals. The first quadrilateral is formed between the upper lip vermillion apex plane at the Cupid's bow peaks (301) and the separation point of the lips (302). The second quadrilateral is formed between the separation point of the lips (302) and the lower lip vermillion apex plane (303). The vertical sides of these two vertically arranged quadrilaterals are related by the ratio 1.0:1.618 (Figure 37).

Four anchor points dictate the location of the four vertical gridlines of Hayduke Facial Grid 2. The first anchor point is located on the right oral commissure (326). The second anchor point is located on the right Cupid's bow peak (327). The third anchor point is located on the left Cupid's bow peak (328). The fourth anchor point is located on the left oral commissure (329). These four anchor points guide the formation of three horizontally arranged quadrilaterals. The quadrilateral formed between the right Cupid's bow peak (327) and left Cupid's bow peak (328) and the quadrilateral formed between the right Cupid's bow peak (327) and right oral commissure (326) have horizontal sides related by the ratio 1.0:1.618. The quadrilateral defined between the right Cupid's bow peak (327) and left Cupid's bow peak (328) and the quadrilateral formed between the left Cupid's bow peak (328) and left oral commissure (329) also have horizontal sides related by the ratio 1.0:1.618.

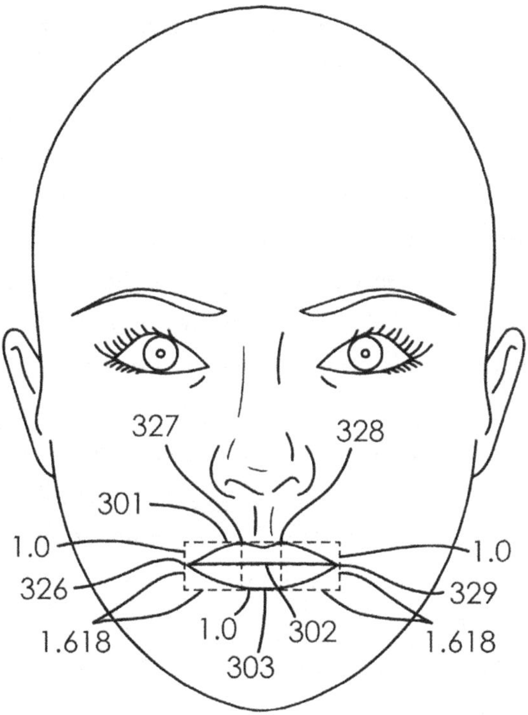

Figure 37. Hayduke Facial Grid 2.

Hayduke Facial Grid 3 (Figure 38) is composed of both horizontally and vertically arranged quadrilaterals. Three anchor points (anatomic landmarks) dictate the location of the horizontal gridlines of this grid. The first anchor point is located on the nasal base plane (313). The second anchor point is located on the upper lip vermillion apex plane at the Cupid's bow peaks (301). The third anchor point is located on the lower lip vermillion apex plane (303). These three anchor points guide the formation of two vertically arranged quadrilaterals. The first quadrilateral is formed between the nasal base plane (313) and the upper lip vermillion apex plane (301). The second quadrilateral is formed between the upper lip vermillion apex plane (301) and the lower lip vermillion apex plane (303). The vertical sides of these two vertically arranged quadrilaterals are related by the ratio 1.0:1.618.

Four anchor points dictate the location for the four vertical gridlines of Hayduke Facial Grid 3. The first anchor point is located on the right Cupid's bow peak (327). The second anchor point is located on the left Cupid's bow peak (328). The third anchor point is located on the left oral commissure (329). The fourth anchor point is located on the right oral commissure (326). These four anchor points guide the formation of three horizontally arranged quadrilaterals. The central quadrilateral between the right Cupid's bow peak (327) and left Cupid's bow peak (328) and the quadrilateral between the right Cupid's bow peak (327) and right oral commissure (326) have horizontal sides related by the ratio 1.0:1.618. The central quadrilateral between the right Cupid's bow peak (327) and left Cupid's bow peak (328) and the quadrilateral between the left Cupid's bow peak (328) and left oral commissure (329) also have horizontal sides related by the ratio 1.0:1.618.

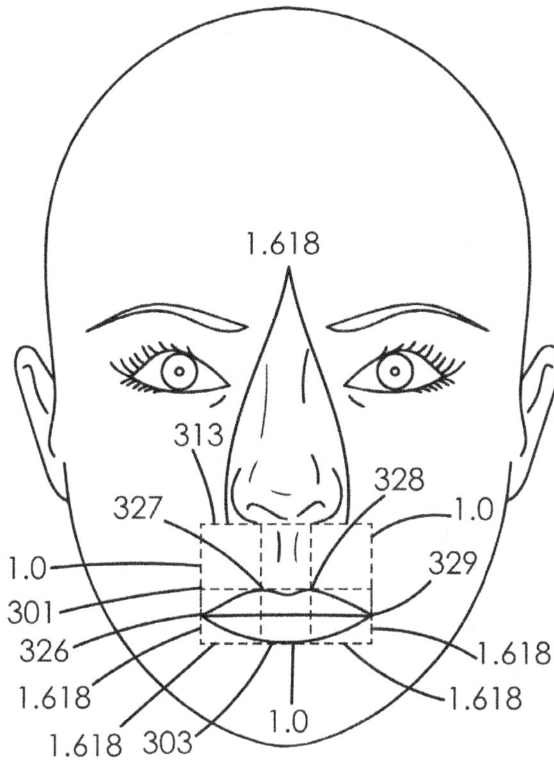

Figure 38. Hayduke Facial Grid 3.

Hayduke Facial Grid 4 (Figure 39) is a grid with three anchor points (anatomic landmarks) that dictate the location of the horizontal gridlines of this grid. The first anchor point is located on the nasal base plane (313). This point dictates the location of the uppermost horizontal gridline. The second anchor point is located on the upper lip vermillion apex plane at the Cupid's bow peaks (301). This point dictates the location of the middle horizontal gridline. The third anchor point is located on the lower lip vermillion apex plane (303). This point dictates the location of the lowermost horizontal gridline. The grid derived from these three anchor points consists of two vertically arranged quadrilaterals. In this overlay, the first quadrilateral is formed between the nasal base plane (313) and the upper lip vermillion apex plane (301). The second quadrilateral is formed between the upper lip vermillion apex plane (301) and the lower lip vermillion apex plane (303). The vertical side of the first quadrilateral is related to the vertical side of the second quadrilateral by the ratio 1.0:1.618.

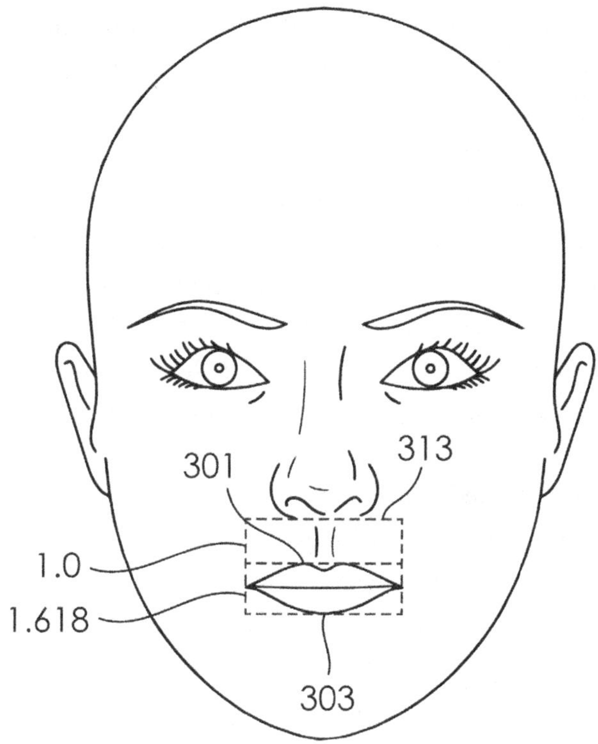

Figure 39. Hayduke Facial Grid 4.

Hayduke Facial Grid 5 (Figure 40) is a grid with three anchor points (anatomic landmarks) that dictate the location of the horizontal gridlines of this grid. The first anchor point is located on the upper lip vermillion apex plane (301). This point dictates the location of the uppermost horizontal gridline. The second anchor point is located on the lower lip vermillion apex plane (303). This point dictates the location of the middle horizontal gridline. The third anchor point is located on the inferior margin of the chin (306). This point dictates the location of the lowermost horizontal gridline. The grid derived from these three anchor points consists of two vertically arranged quadrilaterals. In this overlay, a first quadrilateral is formed between the upper lip vermillion apex plane (301) and the lower lip vermillion apex plane (303). The second quadrilateral is formed between the lower lip vermillion apex plane (303) and the inferior margin of the chin (306). The vertical side of the first quadrilateral is related to the vertical side of the second quadrilateral by the ratio 1.0:1.618.

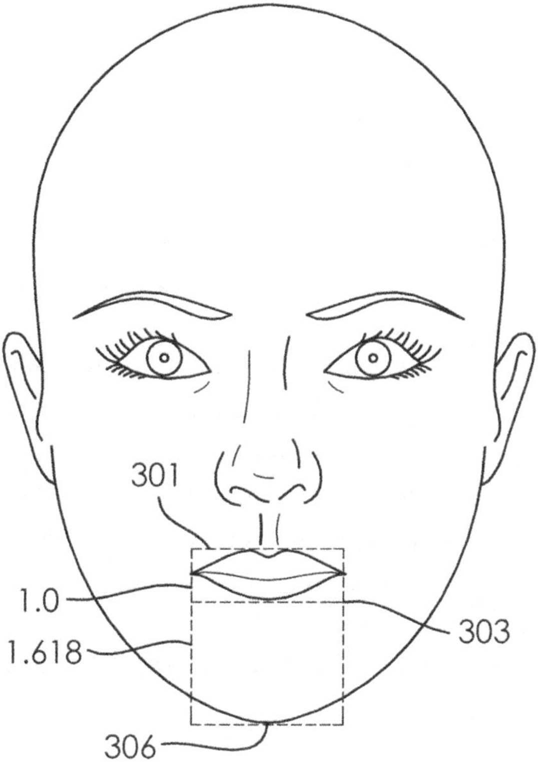

Figure 40. Hayduke Facial Grid 5.

Hayduke Facial Grid 6 (Figure 41) is a grid with three anchor points (anatomic landmarks) that dictate the location of the horizontal gridlines of this grid. The first anchor point is located at the nasal supratip breakpoint (338). This point dictates the location of the uppermost horizontal gridline. The second anchor point is located at the lower lip vermillion apex plane (303). This point dictates the location of the middle horizontal gridline. The third anchor point is located at the inferior margin of the chin (306). This point dictates the location of the lowermost horizontal gridline. The grid derived from these three anchor points consists of two vertically arranged quadrilaterals. In this overlay, the first quadrilateral is formed between the lower lip vermillion apex plane (303) and the inferior margin of the chin (306). The second quadrilateral is formed between the lower lip vermillion apex plane (303) and the nasal supratip breakpoint (338). The vertical side of the first quadrilateral is related to the vertical side of the second quadrilateral by the ratio 1.0:1.618.

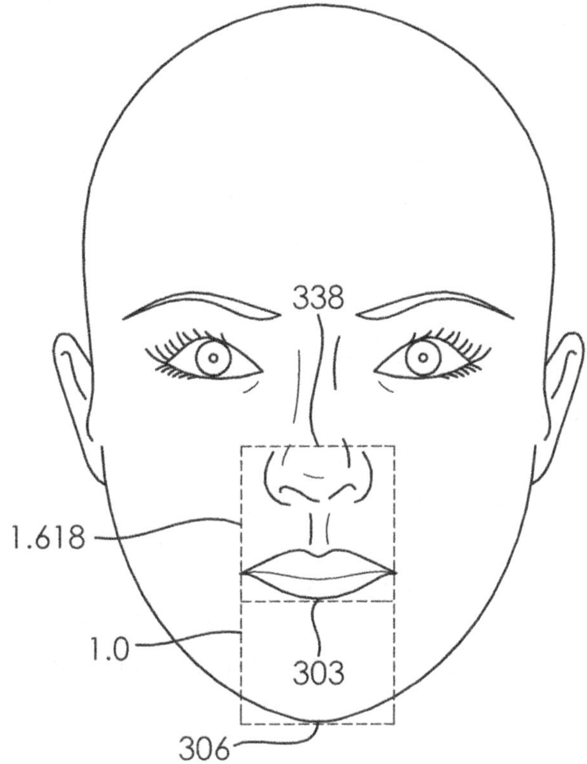

Figure 41. Hayduke Facial Grid 6.

Hayduke Facial Grid 7 (Figure 42) is a grid with three anchor points (anatomic landmarks) that dictate the location of the horizontal gridlines of this grid. The first anchor point is located at the nose supratip breakpoint (338). This point dictates the location of the uppermost horizontal gridline. The second anchor point is located at the upper lip vermillion apex plane (301). This point dictates the location of the middle horizontal gridline. The third anchor point is located at the inferior margin of the chin (306). This point dictates the location of the lowermost horizontal gridline. The grid derived from these three anchor points consists of two vertically arranged quadrilaterals. In this overlay, the first quadrilateral is formed between the upper lip vermillion apex plane (301) and the nose supratip breakpoint (338). The second quadrilateral is formed between the upper lip vermillion apex plane (301) and the inferior margin of the chin (306). The vertical side of the first quadrilateral is related to the vertical side of the second quadrilateral by the ratio 1.0:1.618.

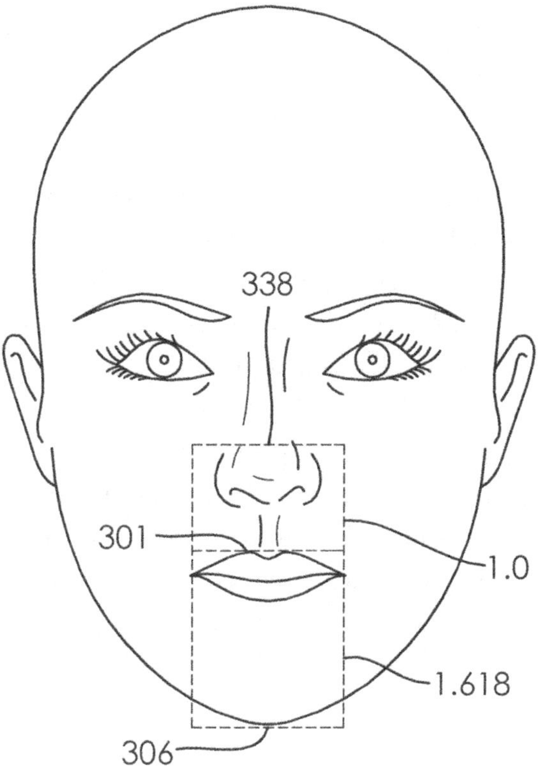

Figure 42. Hayduke Facial Grid 7.

Hayduke Facial Grid 8 (Figure 43) is a grid with three anchor points (anatomic landmarks) that dictate the location of the horizontal gridlines of this grid. The first anchor point is located at the pupillary horizontal plane (305). This point dictates the location of the uppermost horizontal gridline. The second anchor point is located at the nasal base plane (313). This point dictates the location of the middle horizontal gridline. The third anchor point is located at the lower vermillion border (303). This point dictates the location of the lowermost horizontal gridline. The grid derived from these three anchor points consists of two vertically arranged quadrilaterals. In this overlay, a first quadrilateral is formed between the nasal base plane (313) and the lower lip vermillion border (303). The second quadrilateral is formed between the nasal base plane (313) and the pupillary horizontal plane (305). The vertical side of the first quadrilateral is related to the vertical side of the second quadrilateral by the ratio 1.0:1.618.

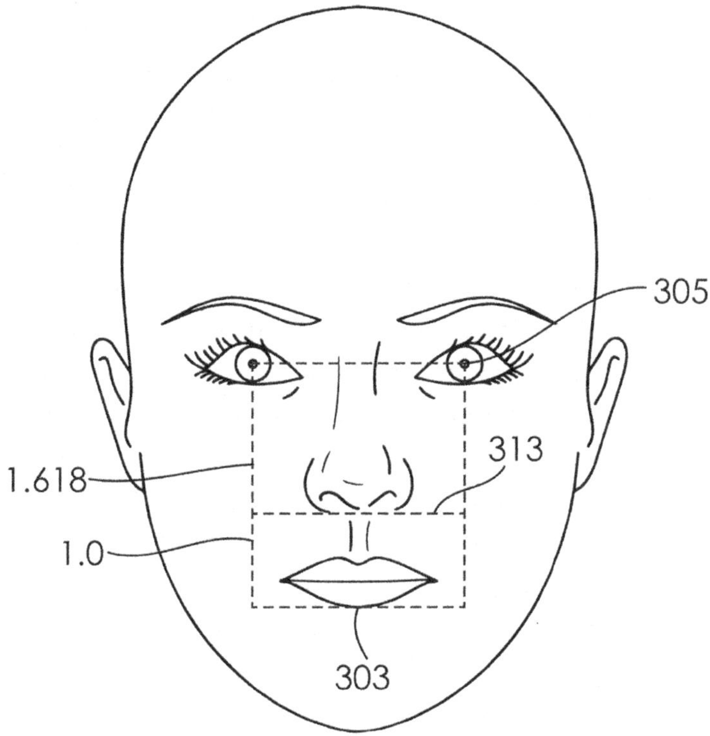

Figure 43. Hayduke Facial Grid 8.

Hayduke Facial Grid 9 (Figure 44) is a grid with three anchor points (anatomic landmarks) that dictate the location of the three horizontal gridlines of this grid. The first anchor point is located at the pupillary horizontal plane (305). This point dictates the location of the uppermost horizontal gridline. The second anchor point is located at a horizontal plane just above the nostril openings (342). This point dictates the location of the middle horizontal gridline. The third anchor point is located at the separation point of the lips (302). This point dictates the location of the lowermost horizontal gridline. The grid derived from these three anchor points consists of two vertically arranged quadrilaterals. In this overlay, the first quadrilateral is formed between the separation point of the lips (302) and the horizontal line just above the nostril openings (342). The second quadrilateral is formed between the horizontal line just above the nostril openings (342) and the pupillary horizontal plane (305). The vertical side of the first quadrilateral is related to the vertical side of the second quadrilateral by the ratio 1.0:1.618.

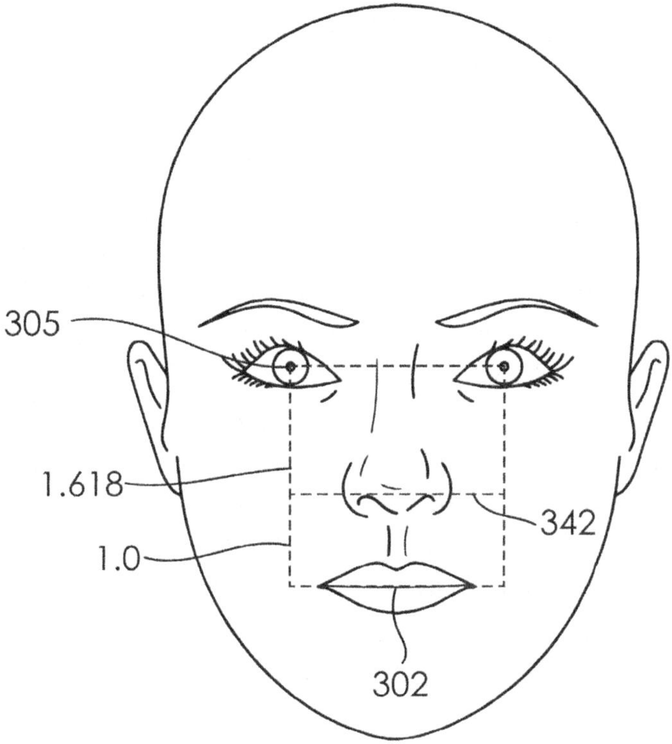

Figure 44. Hayduke Facial Grid 9.

Hayduke Facial Grid 10 (Figure 45) is a grid with three anchor points (anatomic landmarks) that dictate the location of the three horizontal gridlines of this grid. The first anchor point is located at the pupillary horizontal plane (305). This point dictates the location of the uppermost horizontal gridline. The second anchor point is located at the separation point of the lips (302). This point dictates the location of the middle horizontal gridline. The third anchor point is located at the inferior margin of the chin (306). This point dictates the location of the lowermost horizontal gridline. The grid derived from these three anchor points consists of two vertically arranged quadrilaterals. In this overlay, the first quadrilateral is formed between the separation point of the lips (302) and the inferior margin of the chin (306). The second quadrilateral is formed between the separation point of the lips (302) and the pupillary horizontal plane (305). The vertical side of the first quadrilateral is related to the vertical side of the second quadrilateral by the ratio 1.0:1.618.

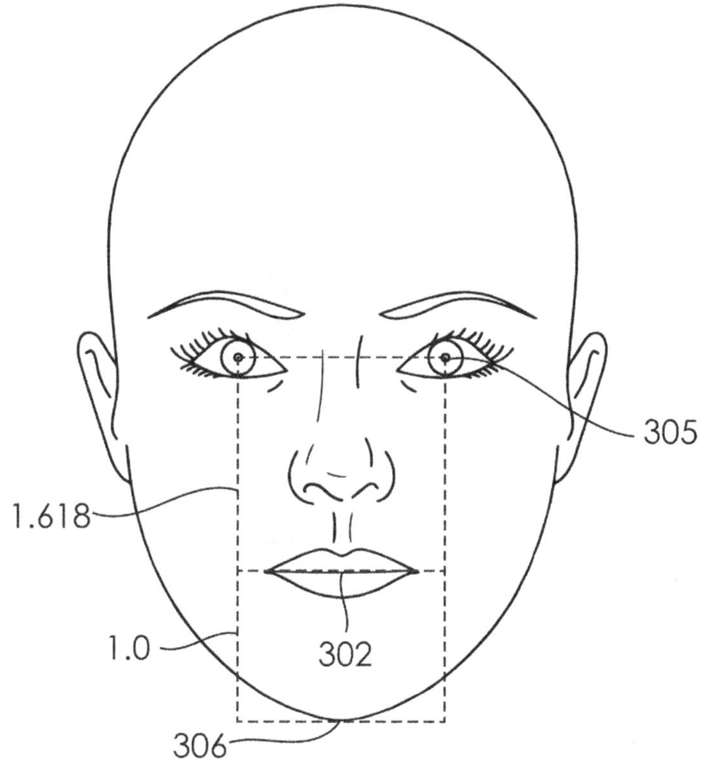

Figure 45. Hayduke Facial Grid 10.

Hayduke Facial Grid 11 (Figure 46) is a grid with three sets of anchor points that dictate the location of the three horizontal gridlines of this grid. The first anchor point is located on the plane at the peaks of the right and left eyebrow arches (307). This point dictates the location of the uppermost horizontal gridline. The second anchor point is located on the upper lip vermillion apex plane (301). This point dictates the location of the middle horizontal gridline. The third anchor point is located at the inferior chin margin (306). This point dictates the location of the lowermost horizontal gridline. In this overlay, the first quadrilateral is formed between the upper lip vermillion apex plane (301) and the inferior chin margin (306). The second quadrilateral is formed between the upper lip vermillion apex plane (301) and the plane at the peaks of the eyebrow arches (307). The vertical side of the first quadrilateral is related to the vertical side of the second quadrilateral by the ratio 1.0:1.618.

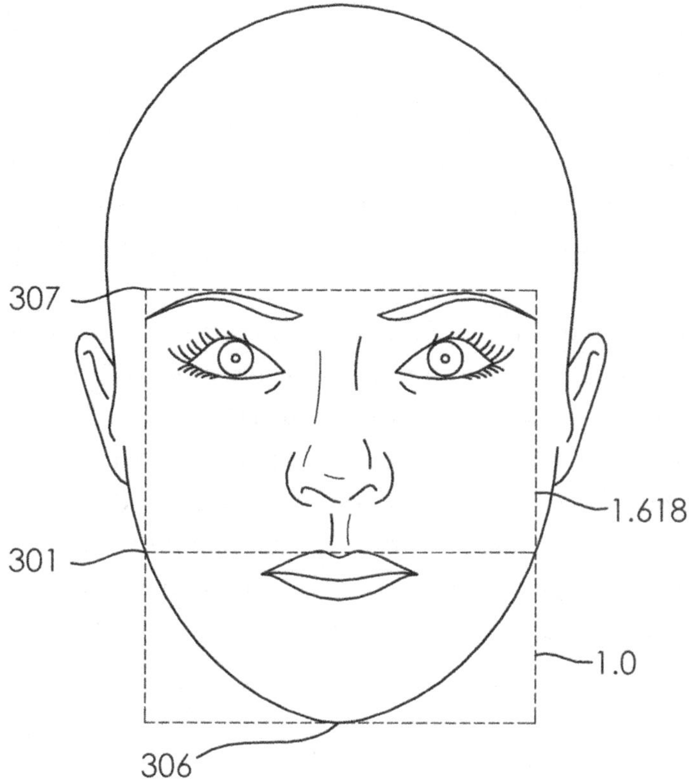

Figure 46. Hayduke Facial Grid 11.

Hayduke Facial Grid 12 (Figure 47) is a grid with four anchor points that dictate the location of the four vertical gridlines of this grid. The first anchor point is located at the right medial canthus (310). The second anchor point is located at the left medial canthus (311). The third and fourth anchor points are located at the inner margins of the right and left nostril openings (346). The distance between the outer vertical sides of this grid is dictated by the distance between the medial canthi. This overlay grid creates an additional relationship wherein the distance between the outer vertical sides of the grid dictates the total base width of the nose. In this overlay, the first quadrilateral is formed between the two inner margins of the nostrils (346). The second and third quadrilaterals are formed between the medial canthus and one inner margin of the nostrils on each side of the first quadrilateral. The horizontal sides of the quadrilaterals are related by the ratio 1.0:1.618.

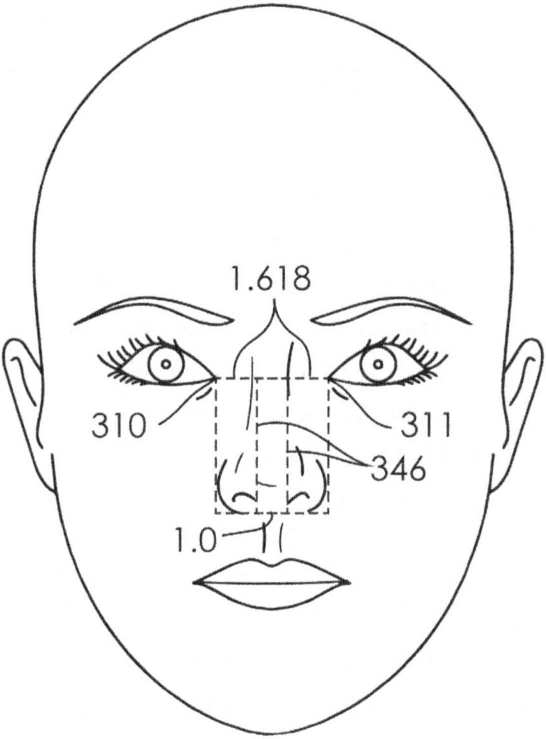

Figure 47. Hayduke Facial Grid 12.

Hayduke Facial Grid 13 (Figure 48) is composed of both horizontally and vertically arranged quadrilaterals. Three anchor points dictate the location of the three horizontal gridlines of this grid. The first anchor point is located at the medial canthal plane (312). The second anchor point is located at the supratip breakpoint of the nose (314). The third anchor point is located at the nasal base plane (313). These three anchor points guide the position of the horizontal gridlines that form two vertically arranged quadrilaterals. The first quadrilateral is formed between the nasal base plane (313) and the supratip breakpoint of the nose (314). The second quadrilateral is formed between the supratip breakpoint of the nose (314) and the medial canthal plane (312). The vertical sides of these two vertically arranged quadrilaterals are related by the ratio 1.0:1.618.

Four anchor points dictate the location of the four vertical gridlines of Hayduke Facial Grid 13. The first anchor point is located at the right medial canthus (310). The second anchor point is located at the left medial canthus (311). The third anchor point is located at the inner margin of the right nostril opening (346). The fourth anchor point is located at the inner margin of the left nostril opening (346). These four anchor points dictate the position of three horizontally arranged quadrilaterals. The horizontal sides of these quadrilaterals are related by the ratio 1.618:1.0, as depicted in Figure 48. The central quadrilateral between the inner margins of the left and right nostril openings (346) and the quadrilateral formed between the inner margin of the left nostril opening and the left medial canthus (311) have horizontal sides related by the ratio 1.0:1.618. The central quadrilateral between the inner margins of the left and right nostril openings (346) and the quadrilateral between the inner margin of the right nostril opening and the right medial canthus (310) are also related by the ratio 1.0:1.618.

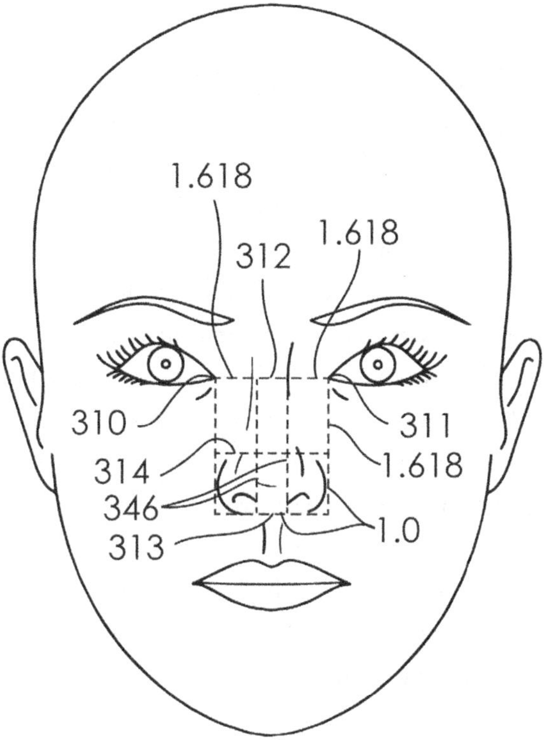

Figure 48. Hayduke Facial Grid 13.

Hayduke Facial Grid 14 (Figure 49) is composed of both horizontally and vertically arranged quadrilaterals. Three anchor points dictate the location of the three horizontal gridlines of this grid. The first anchor point is located at the medial canthal plane (312). The second anchor point is located at the supratip breakpoint of nose (314). The third anchor point is located at the nasal base plane (313). These three anchor points guide the formation of two vertically arranged quadrilaterals. The first quadrilateral is formed between the nasal base plane (313) and the supratip breakpoint of the nose (314). The second quadrilateral is formed between the supratip breakpoint of the nose (314) and the medial canthal plane (312). The vertical sides of these two vertically arranged quadrilaterals are related to each other by the ratio 1.0:1.618.

Four anchor points dictate the location of the four vertical gridlines of Hayduke Facial Grid 14. The first vertical anchor point is located at the midline of the left pupil (308). The second anchor point is located at the midline of the left nostril opening (316). The third vertical anchor point is located at the midline of the right nostril opening (316). The fourth vertical anchor point is located at the midline of the right pupil (309). These four anchor points dictate the position of three horizontally arranged quadrilaterals. The horizontal sides of these three horizontal quadrilaterals are related by the ratio 1.618:1, as depicted in Figure 49. The central quadrilateral located between the midlines of the right and left nostril openings and the quadrilateral located between the midline of the right nostril and the midline of the right pupil have horizontal sides related by the ratio 1.0:1.618. The central quadrilateral located between the midlines of the right and left nostril openings and the quadrilateral located between the midline of the left nostril opening and the midline of the left pupil also have horizontal sides related by the ratio 1.0:1.618.

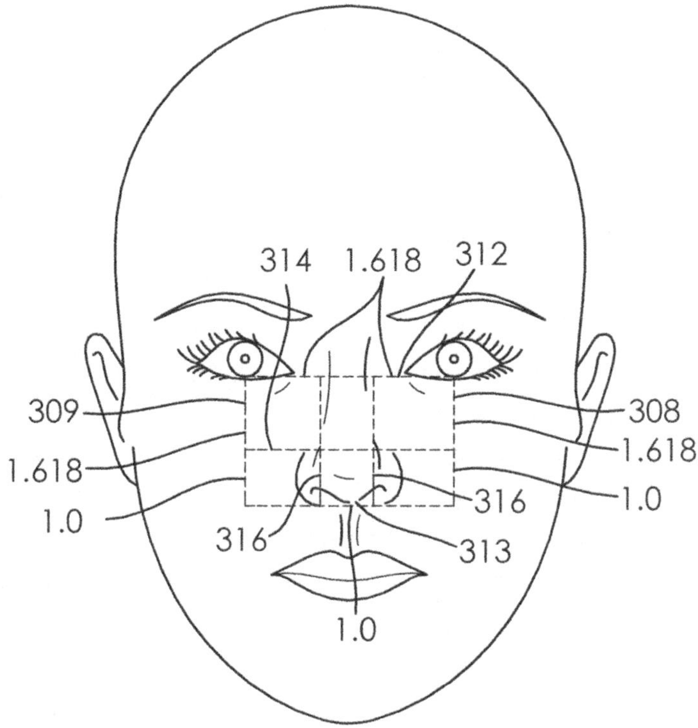

Figure 49. Hayduke Facial Grid 14.

Hayduke Facial Grid 15 (Figure 50) is a grid with six anchor points that dictate the location of the three horizontal gridlines of this grid. The first pair of anchor points is located at the lower eyelid margin (317). The second pair of anchor points is located at the upper eyelid margin (318). The third pair of anchor points is located at the plane at the eyebrow arch peaks (319). The grid derived from these three pairs of anchor points consists of two vertically arranged quadrilaterals. In this overlay, the first quadrilateral is formed between the lower eyelid margin (317) and the upper eyelid margin (318). The second quadrilateral is formed between the upper eyelid margin (318) and the plane at the eyebrow arch peaks (319). The vertical side of the first quadrilateral is related to the vertical side of the second quadrilateral by the ratio 1.0:1.618. Facial symmetry is also tested between the right and left sides of the face with this grid, since two anchor points are involved in each individual horizontal gridline of Hayduke Facial Grid 15. The degree of tilt from a level horizontal plane can be measured between the two anchor points of each horizontal gridline.

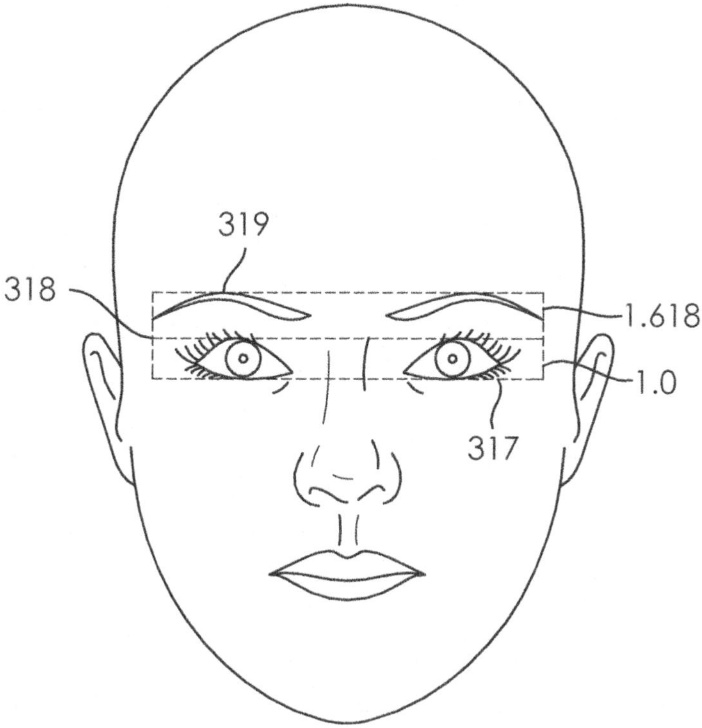

Figure 50. Hayduke Facial Grid 15.

Hayduke Facial Grid 16 (Figure 51) is a grid with three anchor points that dictate the location of the three vertical gridlines of this grid. The first anchor point is located at the outer margin of the temporal process of the zygoma (321). The second anchor point is located at the contralateral (opposite side) medial canthus (311). The third anchor point is located at the contralateral (opposite side) outer margin of the temporal process of the zygoma (320). The grid derived from these three anchor points consists of two horizontally arranged quadrilaterals. In this overlay, a first quadrilateral is formed between the temporal process of the zygoma (320) and the ipsilateral (same side) medial canthus (311). The second quadrilateral is formed between the same canthus that was used in the first quadrilateral and the contralateral (opposite side) temporal process of the zygoma (321). The horizontal sides of these two quadrilaterals are related by the ratio 1.0:1.618. This grid can be reversed (horizontally flipped) and applied to the opposite side of the face. The left medial canthus can be used as the central anchor point for the middle vertical gridline in one version of this grid. The right medial canthus can be used as the central anchor point for the middle vertical gridline in the second version of this grid.

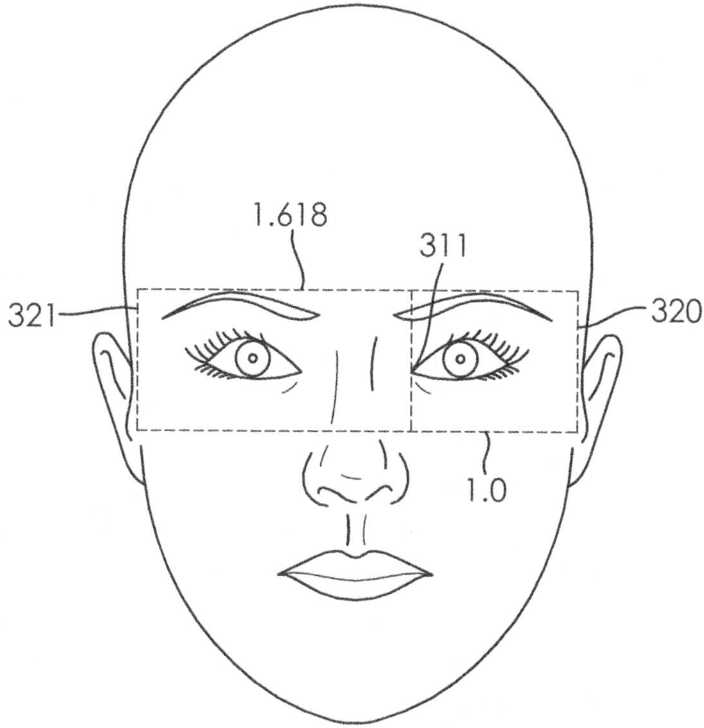

Figure 51. Hayduke Facial Grid 16.

Hayduke Facial Grid 17 (Figure 52) is a grid with three anchor points that dictate the location of the three vertical gridlines of this grid. The first anchor point is located at the temporal process of the zygoma (320). The second anchor point is located at the facial midline (322). The third anchor point is located at the contralateral lateral canthus (323) as related to the temporal process of the zygoma. The grid derived from these three anchor points consists of two horizontally arranged quadrilaterals. The first quadrilateral is formed between the right lateral canthus (323) and the facial midline (322). The second quadrilateral is formed between the facial midline (322) and the left temporal process of the zygoma (320). The horizontal side of the first quadrilateral is related to the horizontal side of the second quadrilateral by the ratio 1.0:1.618. Hayduke Facial Grid 17 can be reversed and applied to the opposite side of the face. The reversed (horizontally flipped) version of this grid would use the right temporal process of the zygoma and the left lateral canthus as anchor points.

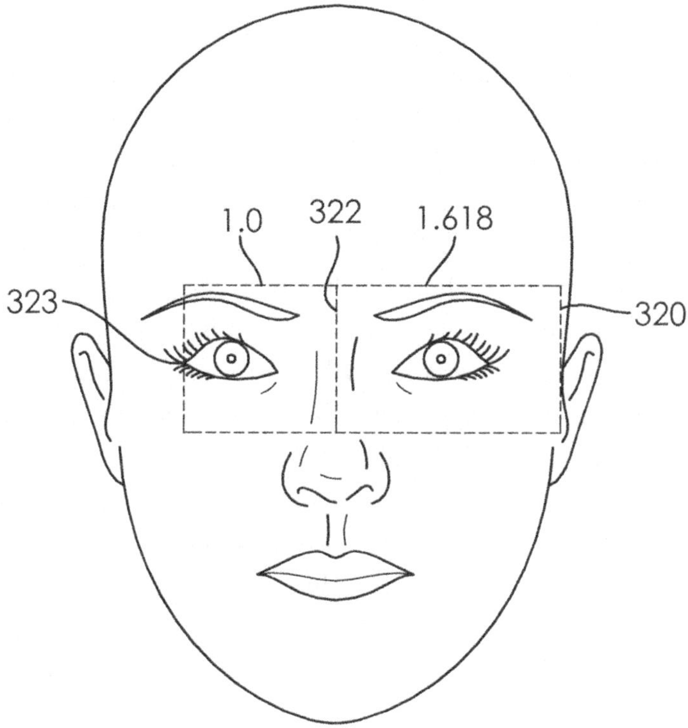

Figure 52. Hayduke Facial Grid 17.

Hayduke Facial Grid 18 (Figure 53) is a grid with three anchor points that dictate the location of the three vertical gridlines of this grid. The first anchor point is located at the temporal process of the zygoma (320). The second anchor point is located at the medial ipsilateral iris margin (324). The third anchor point is located at the facial midline (322). The grid derived from these three anchor points consists of two horizontally arranged quadrilaterals. If the right side of the face is being tested with this grid, the first quadrilateral is formed between the facial midline (322) and the right medial ipsilateral iris margin (324). The second quadrilateral is formed between the right medial ipsilateral iris margin (324) and the right temporal process of the zygoma (320). The horizontal side of the first quadrilateral is related to the horizontal side of the second quadrilateral by the ratio 1.0:1.618. This grid can be reversed (flipped horizontally) to test the left side of the face using the same set of anatomic landmarks that are located on the left side of the face.

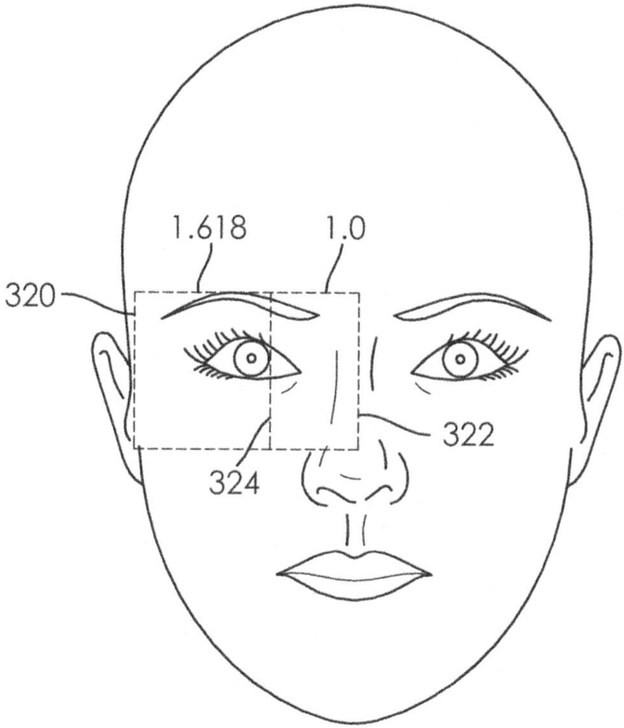

Figure 53. Hayduke Facial Grid 18.

Hayduke Facial Grid 19 (Figure 54) is a grid with three anchor points that dictate the location of the three vertical gridlines of this grid. The first anchor point is located at the temporal process of the zygoma (320). The second anchor point is located at the ipsilateral medial canthus (325). The third anchor point is located at the contralateral medial canthus (311). The grid derived from these three anchor points consists of two horizontally arranged quadrilaterals. If the right side of the face is being tested, the first quadrilateral is formed between the right medial canthus (325) and the left medial canthus (311). The second quadrilateral is formed between the right medial canthus (325) and the right temporal process of the zygoma (320). The horizontal side of the first quadrilateral is related to the horizontal side of the second quadrilateral by the ratio 1.0:1.618. This grid can be reversed (flipped horizontally) to test the left side of the face using the same set of anatomic landmarks that are located on the left side of the face.

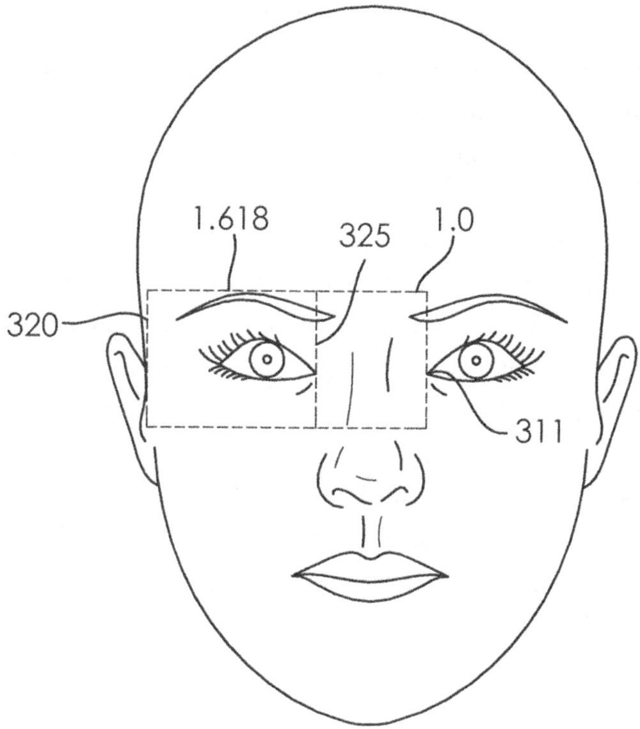

Figure 54. Hayduke Facial Grid 19.

Hayduke Facial Grid 20 (Figure 55) is a grid with three anchor points that dictate the location of the three vertical gridlines of this grid. The first anchor point is located at the temporal process of the zygoma (320). The second anchor point is located at the ipsilateral lateral canthus (330). The third anchor point is located at the ipsilateral pupil (309). The grid derived from these three anchor points consists of two horizontally arranged quadrilaterals. If the right side of the face is being tested, the first quadrilateral is formed between the pupil (309) and the right lateral canthus (330). The second quadrilateral is formed between the right lateral canthus (330) and the right temporal process of the zygoma (320). The horizontal side of the first quadrilateral is related to the horizontal side of the second quadrilateral by the ratio 1.0:1.618. This grid can be reversed (flipped horizontally) to test the left side of the face using the same set of anatomic landmarks that are located on the left side of the face.

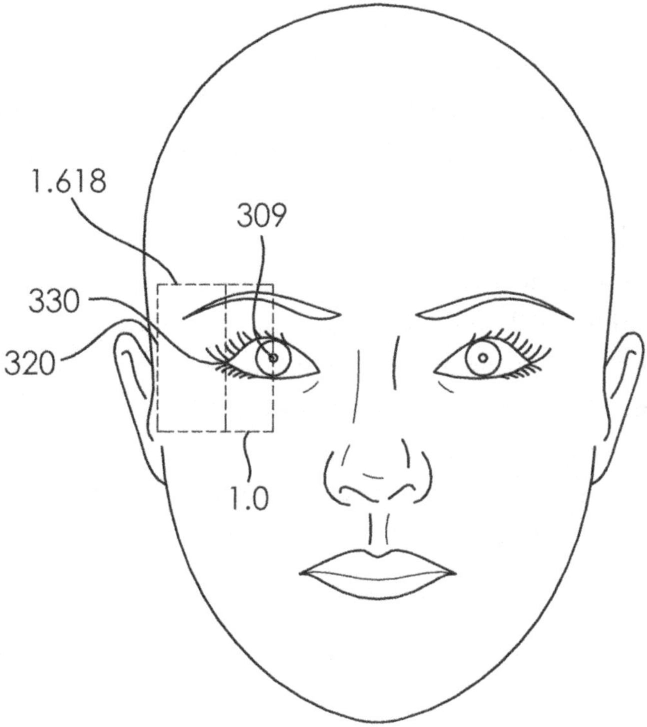

Figure 55. Hayduke Facial Grid 20.

Hayduke Facial Grid 21 (Figure 56) is a grid with three anchor points that dictate the location of the three vertical gridlines of this particular grid. The first anchor point is located at the temporal process of the zygoma (320). The second anchor point is located at the lateral ipsilateral iris margin (331). The third anchor point is located at the ipsilateral medial canthus (310). If the right side of the face is tested, the first quadrilateral is formed between the right medial canthus (310) and the right lateral ipsilateral iris margin (331). The second quadrilateral is formed between the right lateral iris margin (331) and right temporal process of zygoma (320). This grid can be reversed (flipped horizontally) to test the left side of the face using the same set of anatomic landmarks that are located on the left side of the face.

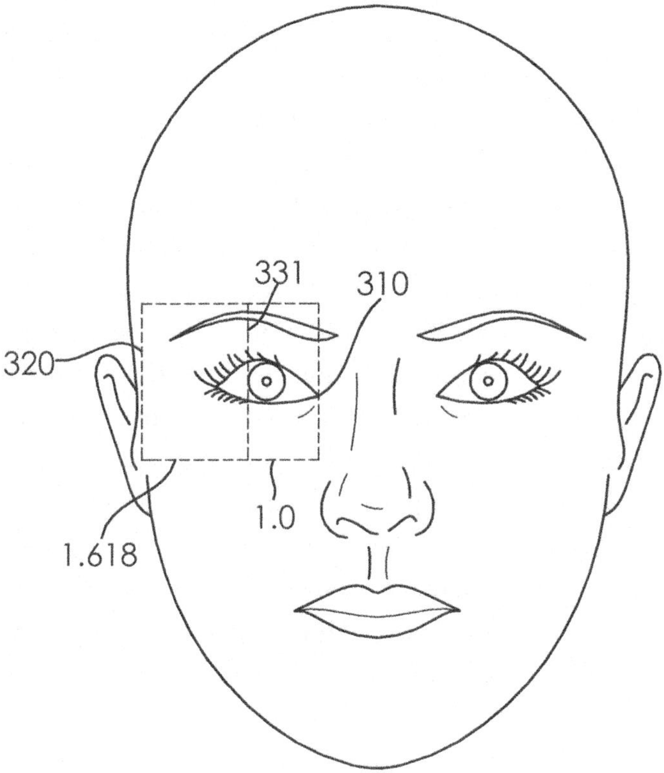

Figure 56. Hayduke Facial Grid 21.

Hayduke Facial Grid 22 (Figure 57) is a grid with three anchor points that dictate the location of the three horizontal gridlines of this grid. The first pair of anchor points is located on the medial canthal plane (312). This pair of anchor points dictates the location of the uppermost horizontal gridline. The second anchor point is located at the supratip breakpoint of nose (314). This point dictates the location of the middle horizontal gridline. The third anchor point is located at the nasal base plane (313). This point dictates the location of the lowermost horizontal gridline. The grid derived from these three anchor points consists of two vertically arranged quadrilaterals. The first quadrilateral is formed between the nasal base plane (313) and the supratip breakpoint of the nose (314). The second quadrilateral is formed between the supratip breakpoint of the nose (314) and the medial canthal plane (312). The vertical side of the first quadrilateral is related to the vertical side of the second quadrilateral by the ratio 1.0:1.618.

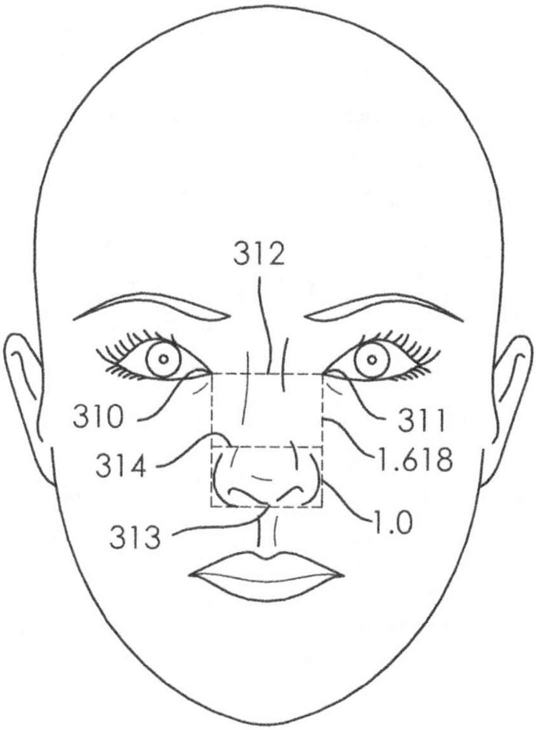

Figure 57. Hayduke Facial Grid 22.

Hayduke Facial Grid 23 (Figure 58) is a grid with four anchor points that dictate the location of the four vertical gridlines of this grid. The first anchor point is located at the midline of the left pupil (308). The second anchor point is located at the midline of the left nostril opening (316). The third anchor point is located at the midline of the right nostril opening (316). The fourth anchor point is located at the midline of the right pupil (309). These four anchor points dictate the formation of three horizontally arranged quadrilaterals. The first quadrilateral is formed between the left and right nostril openings (316). The second quadrilateral is formed between the left nostril opening (316) and the midline of the left pupil (308). The third quadrilateral is formed between the right nostril opening (316) and the midline of the right pupil (309). The horizontal side of the first quadrilateral is related to the horizontal sides of both the second and third quadrilaterals by the ratio 1.0:1.618.

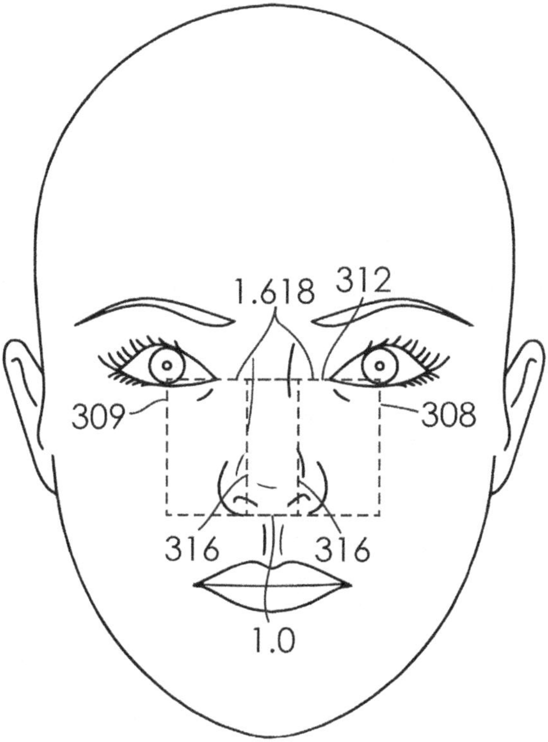

Figure 58. Hayduke Facial Grid 23.

Hayduke Facial Grid 24 (Figure 59) is a grid with three anchor points that dictate the location of the three horizontal gridlines of this grid. The first anchor point is located on the medial canthal plane (312). The second anchor point is located at the supratip breakpoint of the nose (314). The third anchor point is located on the nasal base plane (313). These three anchor points dictate the formation of two vertically arranged quadrilaterals. The first quadrilateral is formed between the nasal base plane (313) and the supratip breakpoint of the nose (314). The second quadrilateral is formed between the supratip breakpoint of the nose (314) and the medial canthal plane (312). The vertical side of the first quadrilateral is related to the vertical side of the second quadrilateral by the ratio 1.0:1.618. The width of Hayduke Facial Grid 24 extends to the right- and left-sided vertical pupillary lines.

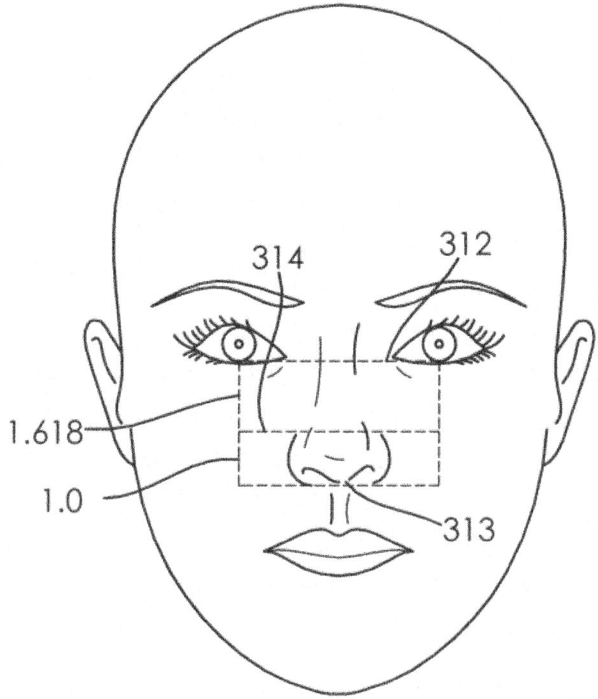

Figure 59. Hayduke Facial Grid 24.

Hayduke Facial Grid 25 (Figure 60) is a grid with four anchor points that dictate the location of the four vertical gridlines of this grid. The first anchor point is located at the right oral commissure (326). The second anchor point is located at the right Cupid's bow peak (327). The third anchor point is located at the left Cupid's bow peak (328). The fourth anchor point is located at the left oral commissure (329). These four anchor points form three horizontally arranged quadrilaterals. The first quadrilateral is formed between the right Cupid's bow peak (327) and left Cupid's bow peak (328). The second quadrilateral is formed between the right Cupid's bow peak (327) and right oral commissure (326). The third quadrilateral is formed between the left Cupid's bow peak (328) and the left oral commissure (329). The horizontal side of the first quadrilateral is related to the horizontal sides of both the second and third quadrilaterals by the ratio 1.0:1.618.

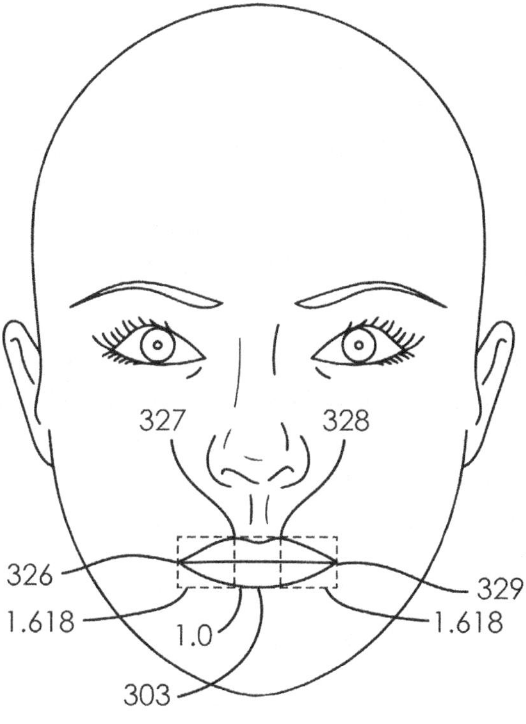

Figure 60. Hayduke Facial Grid 25.

Hayduke Facial Grid 26 (Figure 61) is a right-profile grid with three anchor points that dictate the location of the three vertical gridlines of this grid. The first anchor point is located at the right lateral canthus (332). The second anchor point is located at the nasal radix (333). The third anchor point is located at the anterior margin of the nasal tip (334). The grid derived from these three anchor points consists of two horizontally arranged quadrilaterals. The first quadrilateral is formed between the nasal radix (333) and the anterior margin of the nasal tip (334). The second quadrilateral is formed between the right lateral canthus (332) and the nasal radix (333). The horizontal side of the first quadrilateral is related to the horizontal side of the second quadrilateral by the ratio 1.0:1.618.

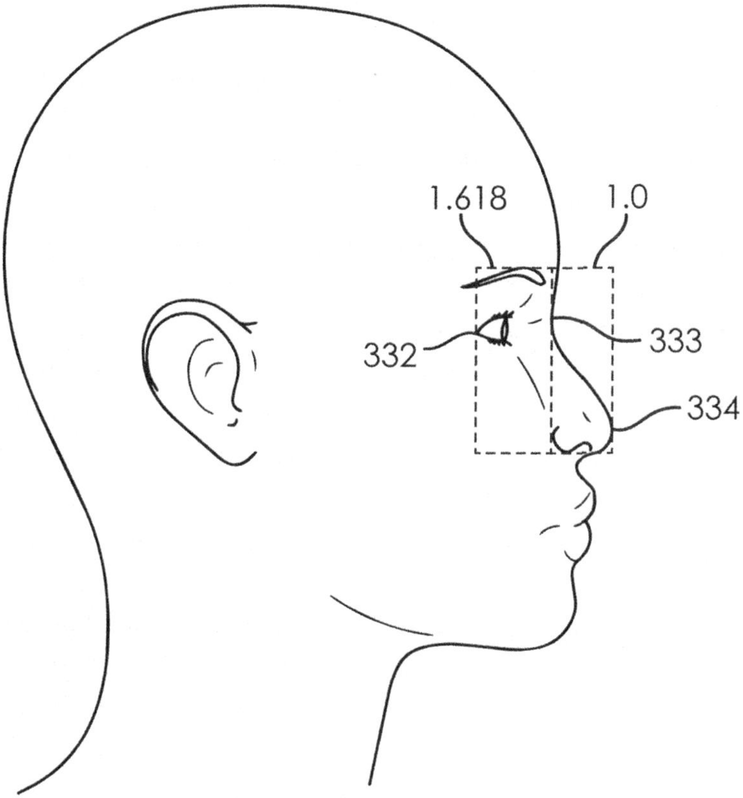

Figure 61. Hayduke Facial Grid 26.

Hayduke Facial Grid 27 (Figure 62) is a right-profile grid composed of both horizontally and vertically arranged quadrilaterals. Three anchor points dictate the location of the three horizontal gridlines of this grid. The first anchor point is located at the peak of the right eyebrow arch (307). The second anchor point is located at the upper lip vermillion apex plane (301). The third anchor point is located at the inferior margin of the chin (306). These three anchor points guide the formation of two vertically arranged quadrilaterals. The first quadrilateral is formed between the inferior margin of the chin (306) and the upper lip vermillion apex plane (301). The second quadrilateral is formed between the upper lip vermillion apex plane (301) and the right eyebrow arch peak (307). The vertical side of the first quadrilateral is related to the vertical side of the second quadrilateral by the ratio 1.0:1.618.

Three anchor points dictate the location of the three vertical gridlines of Hayduke Facial Grid 27. The first vertical anchor point is located at the base of the upper lip philtral dimple (336). The second vertical anchor point is located at the anterior margin of the eyeball (337). The third vertical anchor point is located at the right lateral canthus (332). These three anchor points form two horizontally arranged quadrilaterals. The first quadrilateral is formed between the right lateral canthus (332) and the anterior margin of the eyeball (337). The second quadrilateral is located between the anterior margin of the eyeball (337) and the upper lip philtral dimple (336). The horizontal side of the first quadrilateral is related to the horizontal side of the second quadrilateral by the ratio 1.0:1.618.

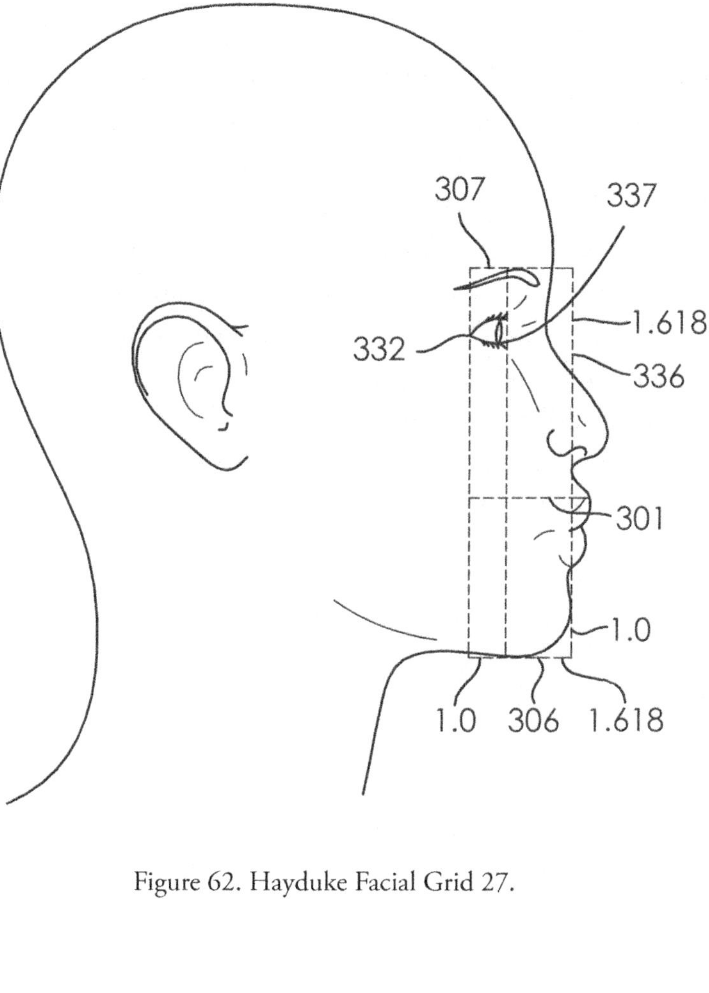

Figure 62. Hayduke Facial Grid 27.

Hayduke Facial Grid 28 (Figure 63) is a right-profile grid with three anchor points that dictate the location of the three horizontal gridlines of this grid. The first anchor point is located at the peak of the right eyebrow arch (307). The second anchor point is located at the upper lip vermillion apex plane (301). The third anchor point is located at the inferior margin of the chin (306). These three anchor points guide the formation of two vertically arranged quadrilaterals. The first quadrilateral is formed between the inferior margin of the chin (306) and the upper lip vermillion apex plane (301). The second quadrilateral is formed between the upper lip vermillion apex plane (301) and the right eyebrow arch peak (307). The vertical side of the first quadrilateral is related to the vertical side of the second quadrilateral by the ratio 1.0:1.618.

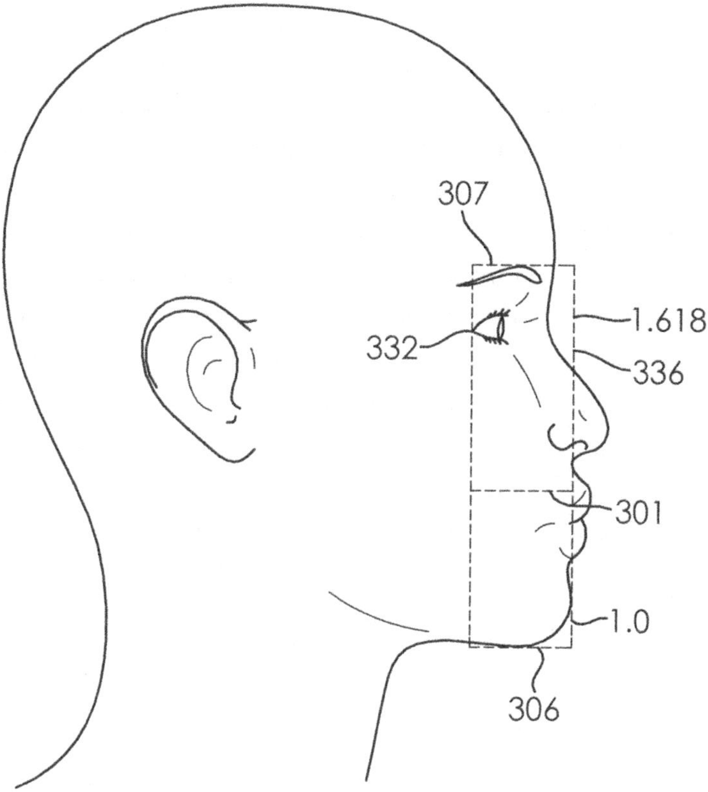

Figure 63. Hayduke Facial Grid 28.

Hayduke Facial Grid 29 (Figure 64) is a right-profile grid with three anchor points that dictate the location of the three vertical gridlines of this grid. The first anchor point is located at the base of the upper lip philtral dimple (336). The second anchor point is located at the anterior margin of the eyeball (337). The third anchor point is located at the lateral canthus (332). These three anchor points guide the formation of two horizontally arranged quadrilaterals. The first quadrilateral is formed between the lateral canthus (332) and the anterior margin of the eyeball (337). The second quadrilateral is formed between the anterior margin of the eyeball (337) and the base of the upper lip philtral dimple (336). The horizontal side of the first quadrilateral is related to the horizontal side of the second quadrilateral by the ratio 1.0:1.618.

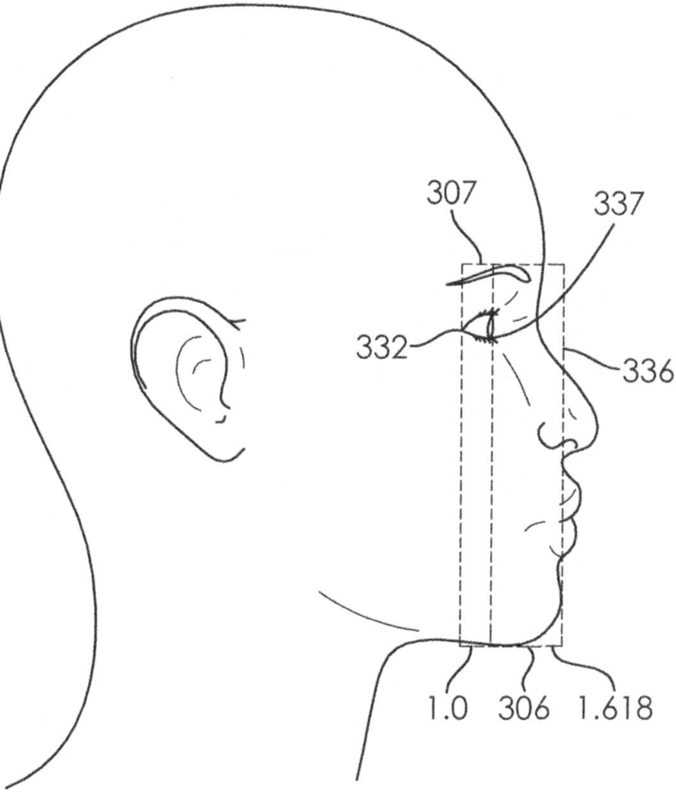

Figure 64. Hayduke Facial Grid 29.

Hayduke Facial Grid 30 (Figure 65) is a left-profile grid with three anchor points that dictate the location of the three vertical gridlines of this grid. The first anchor point is located at the left lateral canthus (332). The second anchor point is located at the nasal radix (333). The third anchor point is located at the anterior margin of the nasal tip (334). The first quadrilateral is formed between the nasal radix (333) and the anterior margin of the nasal tip (334). The second quadrilateral is formed between the left lateral canthus (332) and the nasal radix (333). The horizontal side of the first quadrilateral is related to the horizontal side of the second quadrilateral by the ratio 1.0:1.618.

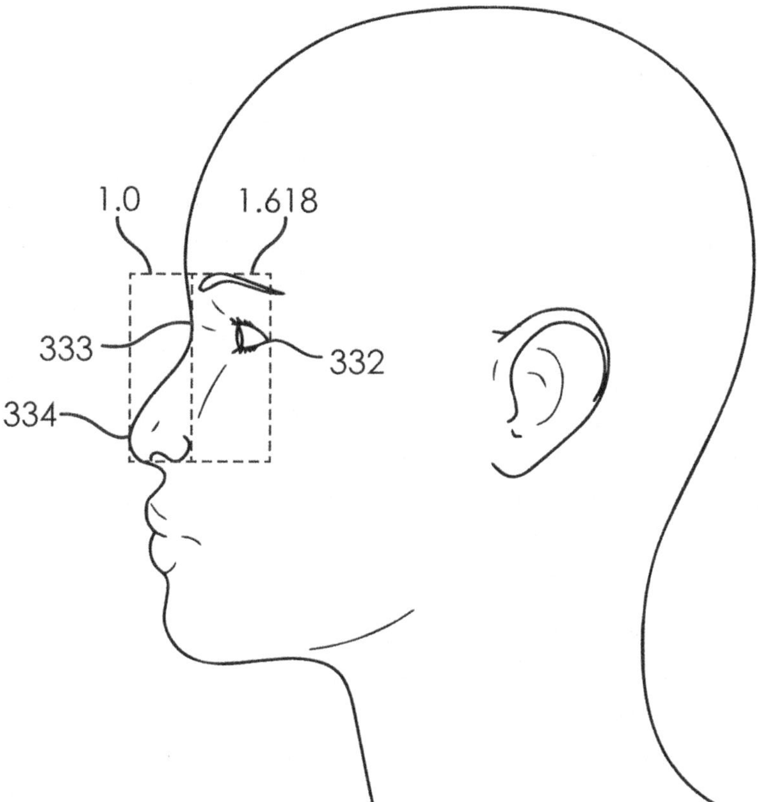

Figure 65. Hayduke Facial Grid 30.

Hayduke Facial Grid 31 (Figure 66) is a left-profile grid composed of both horizontally and vertically arranged quadrilaterals. Three anchor points dictate the location of the three horizontal gridlines of this grid. The first anchor point is located at the peak of the left eyebrow arch (307). The second anchor point is located at the upper lip vermillion apex plane (301). The third anchor point is located at the inferior margin of the chin (306). These three anchor points guide the formation of two vertically arranged quadrilaterals. The first quadrilateral is formed between the inferior margin of the chin (306) and the upper lip vermillion apex plane (301). The second quadrilateral is formed between the upper lip vermillion apex plane (301) and the left eyebrow arch peak (307). The vertical side of the first quadrilateral is related to the vertical side of the second quadrilateral by the ratio 1.0:1.618.

Three anchor points dictate the location of the three vertical gridlines of Hayduke Facial Grid 31. The first anchor point is located at the base of the upper lip philtral dimple (336). The second anchor point is located at the anterior margin of the eyeball (337). The third anchor point is located at the left lateral canthus (332). These three anchor points guide the formation of two horizontally arranged quadrilaterals. The first quadrilateral is formed between the left lateral canthus (332) and the anterior margin of the eyeball (337). The second quadrilateral is formed between the anterior margin of the eyeball (337) and the upper lip philtral dimple (336). The horizontal side of the first quadrilateral is related to the horizontal side of the second quadrilateral by the ratio 1.0:1.618.

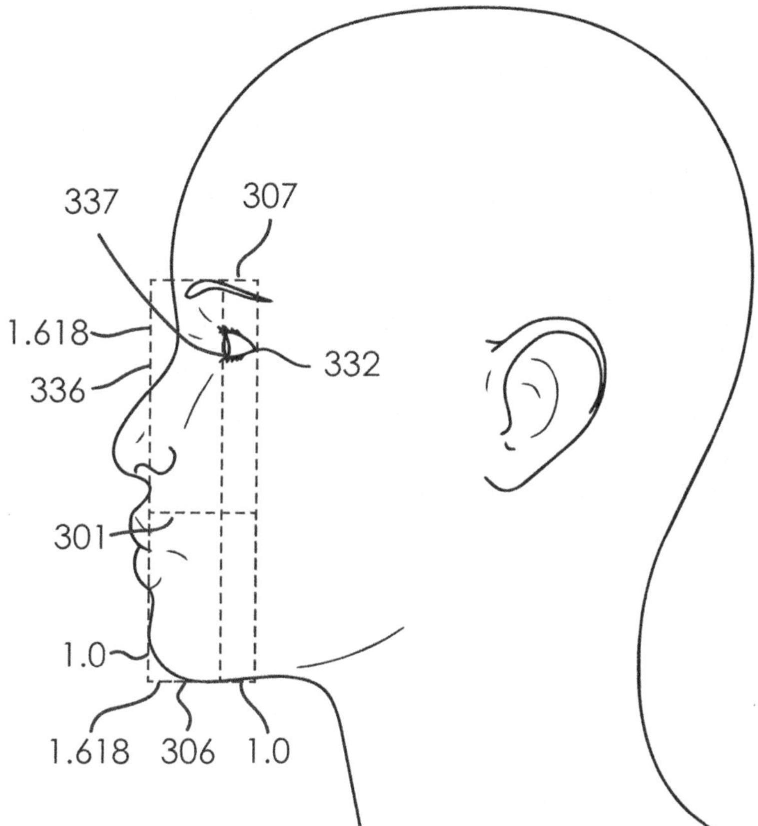

Figure 66. Hayduke Facial Grid 31.

Hayduke Facial Grid 32 (Figure 67) is a left-profile grid with three anchor points that dictate the location of the three horizontal gridlines of this grid. The first anchor point is located at the peak of the left eyebrow arch (307). The second anchor point is located at the upper lip vermillion apex plane (301). The third anchor point is located at the inferior margin of the chin (306). These three anchor points guide the formation of two vertically arranged quadrilaterals. The first quadrilateral is formed between the inferior margin of the chin (306) and the upper lip vermillion apex plane (301). The second quadrilateral is formed between the upper lip vermillion apex plane (301) and the left eyebrow arch peak (307). The vertical side of the first quadrilateral is related to the vertical side of the second quadrilateral by the ratio 1.0:1.618.

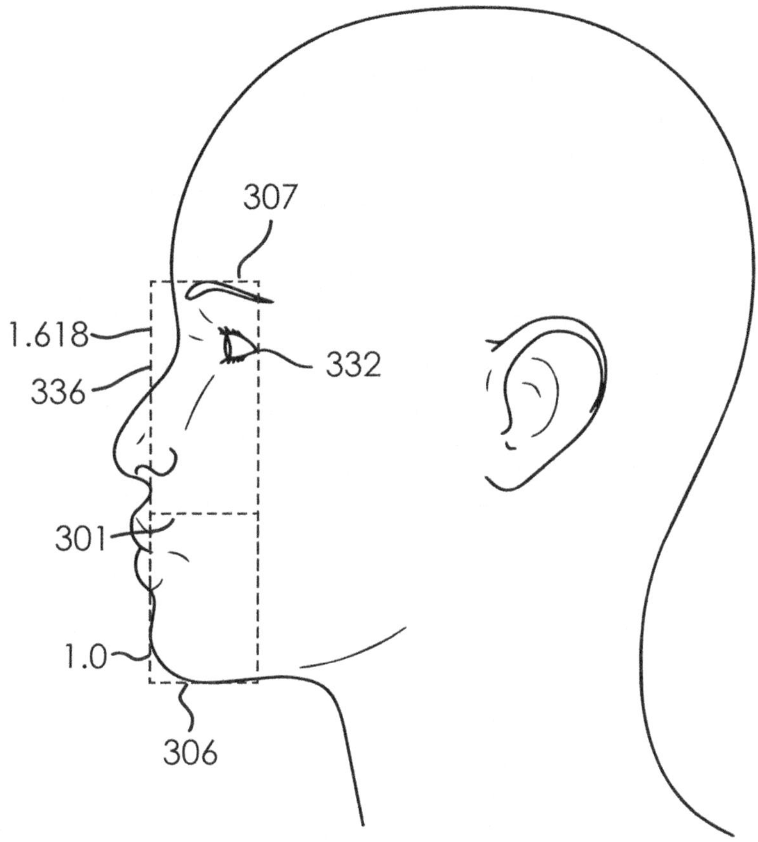

Figure 67. Hayduke Facial Grid 32.

Hayduke Facial Grid 33 (Figure 68) is a left-profile grid with three anchor points that dictate the location of the three vertical gridlines of this grid. The first anchor point is located at the base of the upper lip philtral dimple (336). The second anchor point is located at the anterior margin of the eyeball (337). The third anchor point is located at the lateral canthus (332). These three anchor points form two horizontally arranged quadrilaterals. The first quadrilateral is formed between the lateral canthus (332) and the anterior margin of the eyeball (337). The second quadrilateral is formed between the anterior margin of the eyeball (337) and the base of the upper lip philtral dimple (336). The horizontal side of the first quadrilateral is related to the horizontal side of the second quadrilateral by the ratio 1.0:1.618.

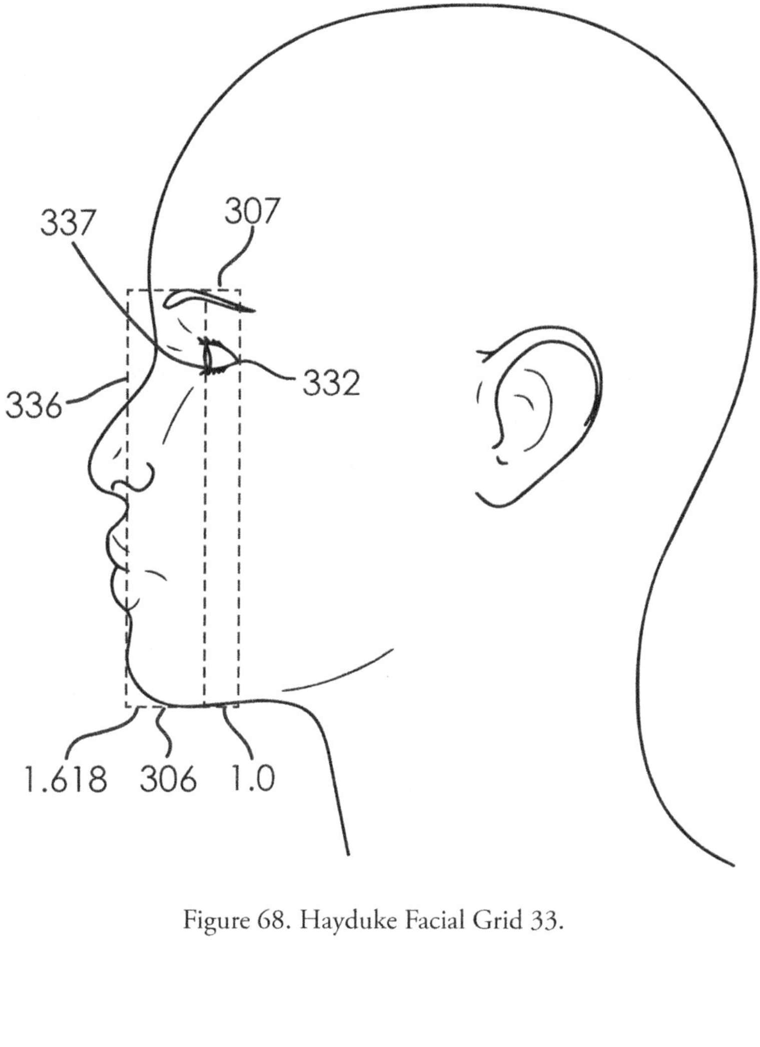

Figure 68. Hayduke Facial Grid 33.

Hayduke Facial Grid 34 (Figure 69) is a right-profile grid with three anchor points that dictate the location of the three vertical gridlines of this grid. The first anchor point is located at the anterior margin of the chin (339). The second anchor point is located at the anterior margin of the eyeball (337). The third anchor point is located at the lateral canthus (332). These three anchor points guide the formation of two horizontally arranged quadrilaterals. The first quadrilateral is formed between the lateral canthus (332) and the anterior margin of the eyeball (337). The second quadrilateral is formed between the anterior margin of the eyeball (337) and the anterior margin of the chin (339). The horizontal side of the first quadrilateral is related to the horizontal side of the second quadrilateral by the ratio 1.0:1.618.

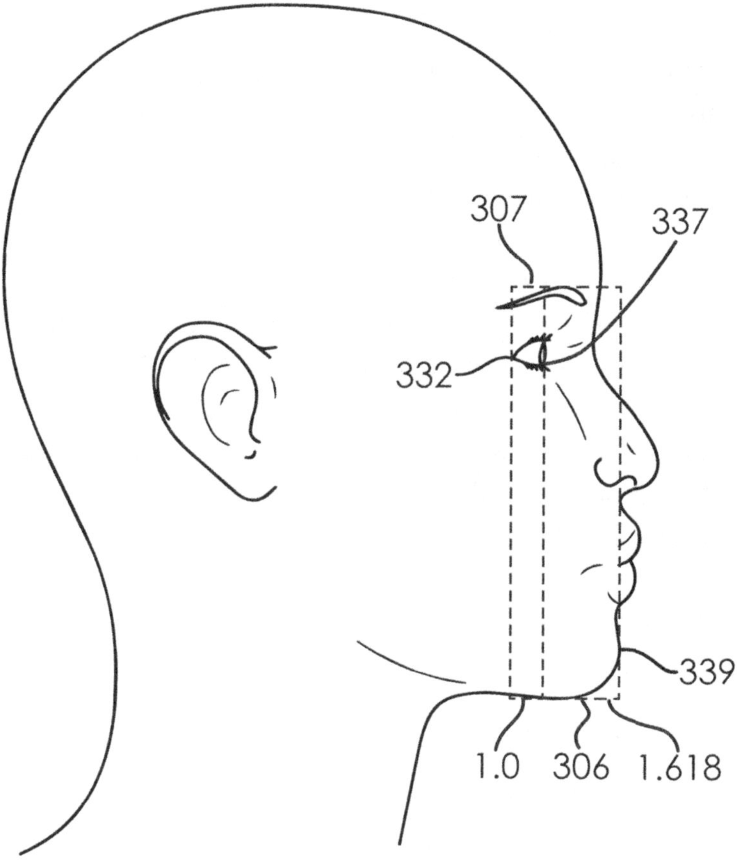

Figure 69. Hayduke Facial Grid 34.

Hayduke Facial Grid 35 (Figure 70) is a left-profile grid with three anchor points that dictate the location of the three vertical gridlines of this grid. The first anchor point is located at the anterior margin of the chin (339). The second anchor point is located at the anterior margin of the eyeball (337). The third anchor point is located at the lateral canthus (332). These three anchor points guide the formation of two horizontally arranged quadrilaterals. The first quadrilateral is formed between the lateral canthus (332) and the anterior margin of the eyeball (337). The second quadrilateral is formed between the anterior margin of the eyeball (337) and the anterior margin of the chin (339). The horizontal side of the first quadrilateral is related to the horizontal side of the second quadrilateral by the ratio 1.0:1.618.

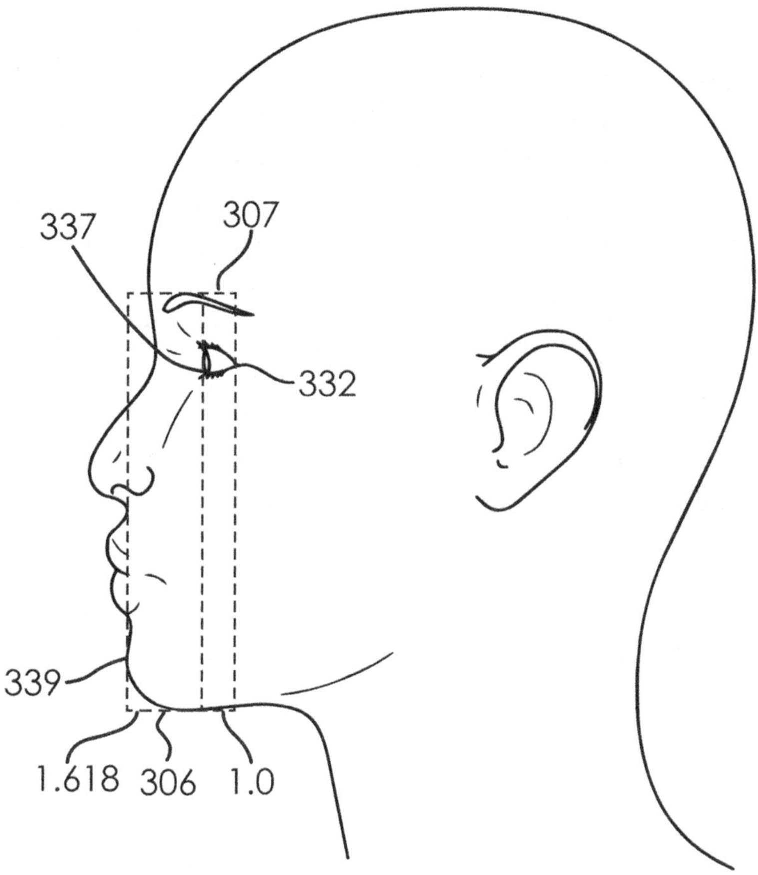

Figure 70. Hayduke Facial Grid 35.

Hayduke Facial Grid 36 (Figure 71) is a right-sided frontal facial grid with three anchor points that dictate the location of the horizontal gridlines of this grid. The first anchor point is located at the right lower eyelid margin (317). The second anchor point is located at the right upper eyelid margin (318). The third anchor point is located at the right eyebrow arch peak (319). The grid derived from these three anchor points consists of two vertically arranged quadrilaterals. The first quadrilateral is formed between the right lower eyelid margin (317) and the right upper eyelid margin (318). The second quadrilateral is located between the right upper eyelid margin (318) and the right eyebrow arch peak (319). The vertical side of the first quadrilateral is related to the vertical side of the second quadrilateral by the ratio 1.0:1.618.

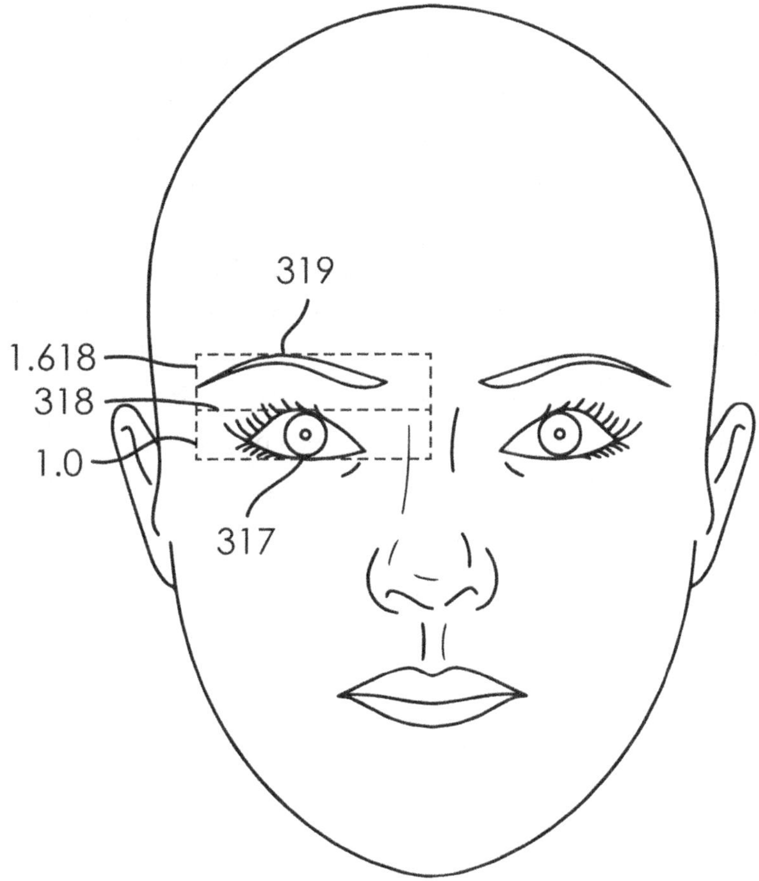

Figure 71. Hayduke Facial Grid 36.

Hayduke Facial Grid 37 (Figure 72) is a left-sided frontal facial grid with three anchor points that dictate the location of the horizontal gridlines of this grid. The first anchor point is located at the left lower eyelid margin (317). The second anchor point is located at the left upper eyelid margin (318). The third anchor point is located at the left eyebrow arch peak (319). The grid derived from these three anchor points consists of two vertically arranged quadrilaterals. In this overlay, the first quadrilateral is formed between the left lower eyelid margin (317) and the left upper eyelid margin (318). The second quadrilateral is located between the left upper eyelid margin (318) and the left eyebrow arch peak (319). The vertical side of the first quadrilateral is related to the vertical side of the second quadrilateral by the ratio 1.0:1.618.

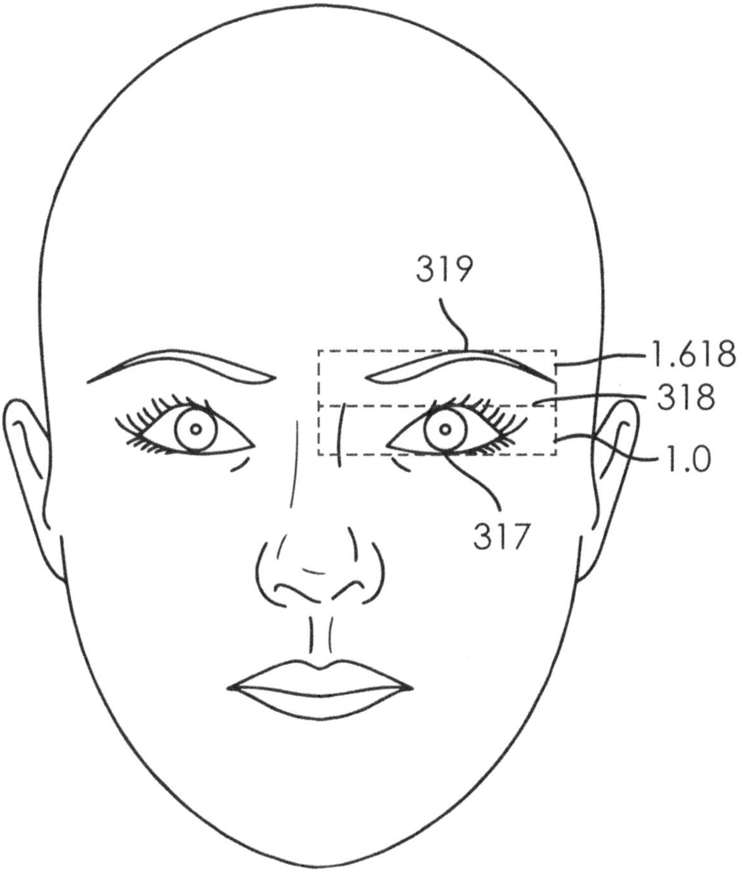

Figure 72. Hayduke Facial Grid 37.

CHAPTER 4

DIVINE BREASTS®

Beauty Analysis of the Human Breast Based on the Golden Ratio

I have designed a system and method that analyzes the surface anatomy of human breasts based on golden ratio anatomic relationships.[1] Overlay digital test grids called Hayduke Breast Grids are used to analyze digital images of human breasts. Hayduke Breast Grids are overlaid on top of images of the client's breasts to see if the anatomic features of the client's breasts conform to the test grids' specifications. My breast analysis methodology is based on golden ratio relationships that are hidden within the physical features of attractive human breasts. Several of the Hayduke Breast Grids also evaluate right- and left-sided breast symmetry.

If the measured distances between the anatomic features of the client's breasts agree with the specific requirements of the particular Hayduke Breast Grid being tested, then a "successful" fit for that particular Hayduke Breast Grid exists. If the anatomic features of the client's breasts don't meet the specifications of the Hayduke Breast Grid being tested, then the client fails that particular Hayduke Breast Grid. The Hayduke Breast Analysis test, which consists of a battery of Hayduke Breast Grids, can be applied to a client's breast images after the required data are inputted into the Divine Breasts® application software.

Image Capture Guidelines

As the first step in my breast analysis methodology, digital images of the client's breasts are uploaded into the Divine Breasts® application software. The most common type of digital images currently used in my plastic surgery practice are high-resolution, two-dimensional, digital still photographs taken with an interchangeable-lens, high-resolution digital camera. Three-dimensional digital photographs and digital video images are other types of digital images that can be applied to my breast analysis methodology.

Proper clinical breast photography requires that the client's body jewelry be totally removed. Clothing should be removed to allow full exposure of the entire breasts, shoulders, and lower abdomen. Pants and underwear need to be lowered to the pubic region to fully expose the lower abdomen. If the client has a large amount of overhanging lower abdominal skin and fat, then their underwear and pants should be lowered even farther to prevent any distortion of the umbilicus (belly button) by their clothing. The lower abdominal skin and fat should be allowed to hang freely without any restriction or distortion by clothing. Hair in females should be pulled back behind the shoulders in a ponytail to avoid obscuring shoulder anatomy. Images should be framed from just above the pubic area to the middle of the neck. The client's arms should be held in a simple, relaxed, natural position at the sides of their body. This avoids causing any unnatural distortion (stretching) of the breasts' appearance secondary to arm positioning. Orienting the camera vertically (portrait orientation) will allow inclusion of the required chest and abdominal anatomy. Photography of the client's face should be specifically avoided within the breast photographs. Breast photographs required for the Divine Face® application software include frontal, right profile, right three-quarter (right oblique), left profile, and left three-quarter (left oblique) poses.

Each breast digital image should ideally include a certified metric ruler within the actual image itself. For clinical use, I recommend that health care professionals purchase a certified metric ruler that possesses a certificate of accuracy traceable to the National Institute of Standards and Technology (NIST). This assures that the ruler within the image (with its own unique serial number) actually passed tests for accuracy. I recommend partially inserting a small portion (about one third) of a certified metric ruler inside the client's pants or underwear in such a way that the image taken captures the ruler in each pose. The metric graduation marks (lines) within the ruler should be clearly visible and sharply in focus when the image is taken. Non-glare surface rulers are best for clinical photography. Bright photographic light flash bursts may obscure the graduation marks of highly reflective metallic rulers. The ruler will require repositioning within the pants or underwear for each individual pose in order to keep the graduation marks clearly visible within the image. The ruler should not obscure the umbilicus at any time.

The camera's lens should be positioned on the exact same plane as the client's breasts. Ideally, a tripod should be used to eliminate camera movement during digital image capture. To minimize camera-induced distortion of breast anatomy, the digital image properties for breast photography should be equivalent to those taken with a 50 to 60 mm focal length lens on a single-lens reflex 35 mm film camera.[2] This focal length recommendation for clinical breast photography was agreed on by the Clinical Photography Committee of the Plastic Surgery Education Foundation. In the age of digital cameras, the crop factor of the specific digital camera's image sensor must be known in order to choose the proper digital camera lens focal length to achieve this goal. Use of a high-quality digital camera, such as a digital single-lens reflex (DSLR) camera or digital mirrorless camera with interchangeable lens capability allows one to easily use the proper lens focal length required for clinical breast photography. It's recommended that a female assistant always be present in the photography room if a male is taking the breast photographs.

The ideal lighting for capturing clinical breast images is "flat lighting" that doesn't create any significant unnatural dark shadows on the client's breasts, abdomen, or background. Studio lighting with multiple lights is preferred. Two main lights at 45-degree angles to the client combined with background lighting to eliminate shadows in the background is highly recommended.

For single light-source situations, the camera's flash should not be pointed directly at the client's breasts but rather bounced off the ceiling to help diffuse the light. This "bounce flash" technique works well in a room with a low white ceiling. Another approach is to use a plastic flash diffuser snapped directly over the camera's flash. This device is a thin, white, plastic cap that gently scatters the light from the camera's flash to eliminate dark shadows on the subject. Strong dark shadows on the breasts obscure anatomic detail required for a true, high-quality breast analysis. White balancing should also be performed to capture the most realistic colors if color images are taken. The resolution of the digital images should be as high as the digital camera and technology allow.

Basic client intake information as well as specific measurements obtained directly from the client's physical examination are manually entered into the client database section of the Divine Breasts® application software. Males who take the physical measurements of the client's breasts should always have a female assistant present in the room during the physical examination (measurement) process. Scanned or photographed documents—such as signed consent forms, model image releases, and copies of the client's identification cards—can also be uploaded into the database section of the Divine Breasts® application.

Labeling Breast Images with Anatomic Markers

The next step in the analysis involves accurate placement of overlay markers (digital dots) onto specific anatomic breast landmarks of the captured digital images. The breast photographs have several automatic anatomic landmarks immediately superimposed upon the uploaded images via computer vision technology. In addition to these automatically generated anatomic landmarks, several other anatomic landmark markers require manual repositioning by the Divine Breasts® application user. The application user refers to a reference image with properly placed anatomic overlay markers (digital dots) to guide the manual landmark repositioning process on the client's breast images being tested. The reference image for each pose is located on the left side of the computer screen, while the client's uploaded image is located on the right side of the computer screen. Each breast anatomic landmark overlay marker (digital dot) must be fine-tuned by the user and repositioned in the proper resting position. The final approved resting position of the anatomic landmark overlay marker is then formally confirmed by the user in order to proceed to the next step of the analysis. Once the anatomic landmark position is approved by the user, the digital anatomic landmark dots change color from red to green to give visual confirmation that the landmark position was formally approved.

The measurement scale is then set using the "set scale" tool within the Divine Breasts® application. The measurement scale is the reference scale that allows the Divine Breasts® application to measure accurate distances—down to millimeters—within the captured digital images. Measurement scale setting can be achieved by using either the image of the metric ruler that was included in each original breast image or via specific anatomic measurements derived from physical examination of the client's breasts. After achieving proper measurement scale settings for all the poses of the breast images, the clients' breast images can now be tested with a battery of Hayduke Breast Grids.

Analyzing Breast Images with Hayduke Breast Grids

For breast analysis, multiple Hayduke Breast Grids are used to analyze the client's digital breast images. At this point, the measurement scale has been set for all the poses and all the anatomic landmarks on the client's images have been marked with overlay markers.

Each Hayduke Breast Grid is based on the relationship of the golden ratio within the grid to a specific set of defined breast anatomic landmarks. Each individual grid in my series is composed of a unique set of specified anatomic landmarks that define the exact gridline location within the grid. The location of the golden ratio anatomic relationship, based on the gridlines, is unique to each individual overlay grid. Each breast grid is also assigned a specific number for identification purposes—Hayduke Breast Grid 1, Hayduke Breast Grid 2, Hayduke Breast Grid 3, etc.

As an example, Hayduke Breast Grid 5 (Figure 73) is a simple breast overlay grid in my series of breast grids. Hayduke Breast Grid 5 has three anatomic landmarks (anchor points) that dictate the location of the three horizontal gridlines of this grid. The first anatomic landmark is located at the base of the jugular suprasternal notch (labeled 401 in Figure 73). This landmark dictates the location of the uppermost horizontal gridline. The second anatomic landmark is located at the superior margin of the right areola (labeled 404 in Figure 73). This landmark dictates the location of the middle horizontal gridline. The third anatomic landmark is located at the inferior margin of the right breast (labeled 416 in Figure 73). This landmark dictates the location of the lowermost horizontal gridline. Two vertically arranged quadrilaterals are formed. In this overlay, the first quadrilateral is formed between the jugular suprasternal notch (401) and the superior border of the right areola (404). The second quadrilateral is formed between the superior border of the right areola (404) and the inferior margin of the right breast (416). The lengths of the vertical sides of these two quadrilaterals are related by a ratio that reduces to 1.618:1.0 (Figure 73).

In the schematic of Hayduke Breast Grid 5 (Figure 73), the vertical side of the upper quadrilateral is labeled "1.618" with a curly bracket. The vertical side of the lower quadrilateral is labeled "1.0". This ratio is derived from measurements of the vertical sides of the two vertically arranged quadrilaterals that make up this grid. For a client's breast to be scored as a "successful" fit of Hayduke Breast Grid 5, the client's anatomic structures would need to be related to each other in such a way that the measured lengths of the grid's two vertical side components would reduce to a ratio of 1.618:1.0. If the client's nipple is positioned very low on the breast or if the client's entire breast is extremely long and droopy, then the reduced ratio derived from the lengths of the vertical sides of the two vertically arranged quadrilateral components wouldn't equal 1.618:1.0. In that situation, this particular grid would be scored as a "failed" grid. If the anatomic features of the client's breast that dictate the gridlines are indeed related to each other by a ratio of 1.618:1.0, then a golden ratio relationship exists between those particular anatomic features. In that case, Hayduke Breast Grid 5 would be scored as a "successful" fit, and the client would receive a point toward the total score of the Hayduke Breast Analysis test.

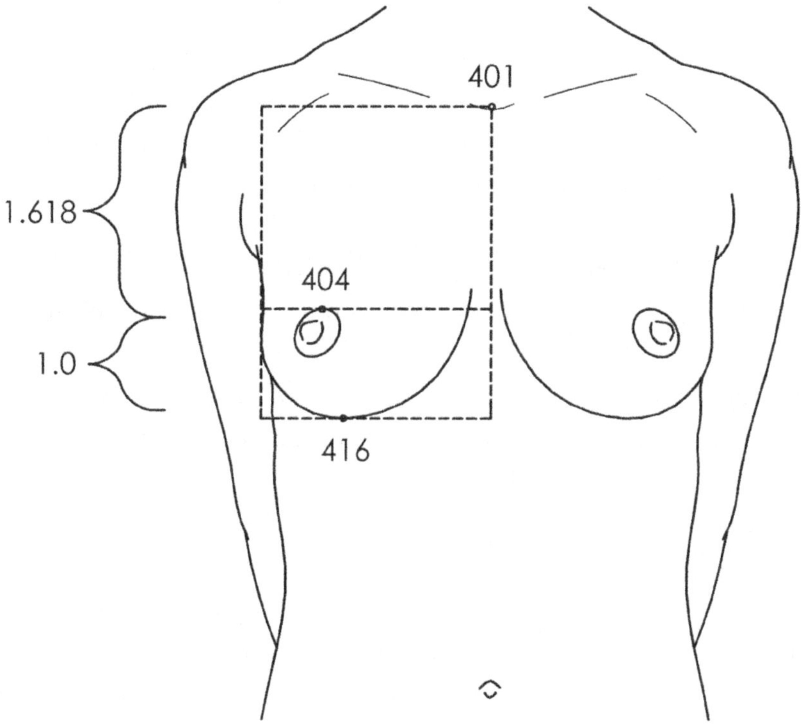

Figure 73. Hayduke Breast Grid 5.

Another example of a simple breast grid within my breast grid series is Hayduke Breast Grid 10 (Figure 74). Hayduke Breast Grid 10 is a grid with three anatomic landmarks (anchor points) that dictate the location of the three vertical gridlines of this grid. The first anchor point is located at the medialmost (inner) margin of the left breast (labeled 403 in Figure 74). The second anchor point is located at the medial (inner) border of the left areola (labeled 412 in Figure 74). The third anchor point is located at the lateralmost (outer) margin of the left breast (labeled 415 in Figure 74). Two horizontally arranged quadrilaterals are formed. In this overlay, the first quadrilateral is formed between the medial margin of the left breast (403) and the medial border of the left areola (412). The second quadrilateral is formed between the medial border of the left areola (412) and the lateralmost margin of the left breast (415). In order to be scored as a "successful" grid, the lengths of the horizontal sides of these two quadrilaterals should reduce to a ratio of 1.618:1.0, as depicted in the schematic (Figure 74). If the client's breast being tested has an areola (nipple) that's in an unattractive position, such as shifted over strangely to either side of the breast, then the reduced ratio derived from the measured lengths of the horizontal sides of the two quadrilaterals won't equal 1.618:1.0. In that situation, Hayduke Breast Grid 10 would be scored as a failed grid.

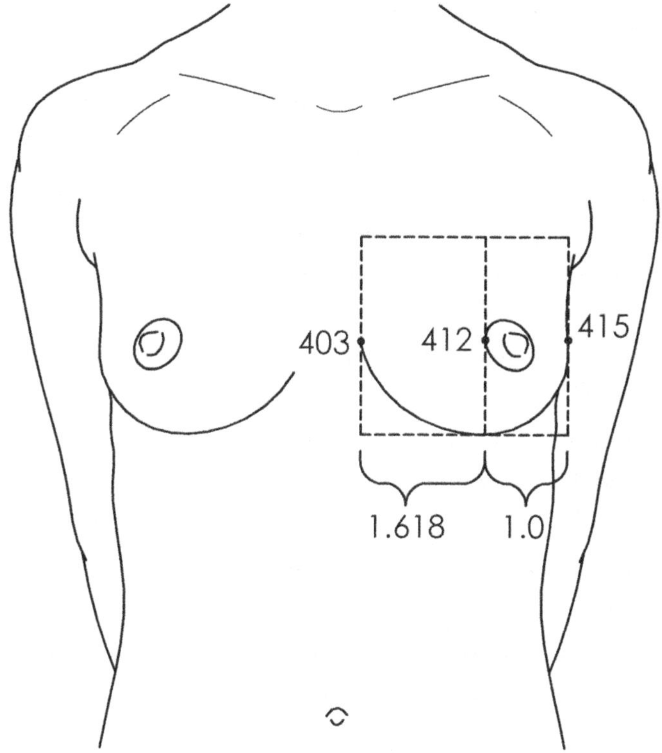

Figure 74. Hayduke Breast Grid 10.

Generating a Hayduke Breast Analysis Test Score Report

After choosing which specific Hayduke Breast Grids to test, a Hayduke Breast Analysis test score report may be requested by the Divine Breasts® application user. The Hayduke Breast Analysis test score report displays the names of the successful grids and failed grids from the specific grids chosen for testing. These results are displayed as "section" scores (frontal, right profile, left profile etc.) as well as a "total" score for all the sections (poses) combined. The total Hayduke Breast Analysis test score is displayed as a percentage of successful grids as well as a numerical fraction of successful grids to total grids tested. In addition, the percentage of successful grids and the ratios of successful grids to failed grids are displayed individually for each of the sections (frontal, right profile, left profile, etc.).

For each section (pose), the specific grid names of the successful grids and failed grids are displayed as well as the "degree of grid fit" of each grid. The degree of grid fit, reported in parenthesis after the specific successful grid name, reports how close a successful grid was to an absolutely perfect fit (range of 1 to 1000, with 1000 reflecting an absolutely perfect grid fit). The "grid ratio offset" setting can also be adjusted by the application user. The grid ratio offset setting reflects how much the grids can vary from an absolutely perfect fit of the specified 1.0:1.618 relationships within the grids tested (expressed as a percentage) and still be considered a successful grid fit. The other setting that can be adjusted by the Divine Breasts® application user is the "grid rotational offset setting." The grid rotational offset setting dictates the specific degree of rotational tilt within a grid that is allowed for grids to still be scored as successful. This allows for some unintentional tilt (rotation) in the client's image at the time of image capture, as well as for minor anatomic asymmetry. At the end of the session, a Divine Breasts® Hayduke Breast Analysis "score report" can be printed out. The score report can be given to the client as a hard copy or saved in the patient's clinical file (chart). This score report includes identifying information such as the client's name, image (photograph) date, date of birth, client's age at the time of breast image capture, height, and weight. The client's data are also stored automatically at the end of the test within the Divine Breast® application software. Saved data include the confirmed anatomic landmark positions on all of the client's uploaded digital images.

Additions and revisions to the design of individual Hayduke Breast Grids and to the Divine Breast® application software are constantly being implemented to achieve maximal analytic quality of the Hayduke Breast Analysis test.

(Detailed technical descriptions of each individual Hayduke Breast Grid are presented in the section below. Some readers may choose to skip this technical section and proceed to the next chapter.)

Technical Specifications of Individual Hayduke Breast Grids

Hayduke Breast Grids and the specific combination of anatomic landmarks involved in each grid's design are the core elements of my system and method of analyzing human breast anatomy (U.S. Patent application number 16593126). Hayduke Breast Grid designs included in the current version of the Hayduke Breast Analysis are detailed below. The breast schematics illustrate a simplified general anatomic layout of the individual golden ratio breast grids; however, the schematics do not actually harbor the 1.618:1.0 ratio within the illustrations' drawn dimensions. Written descriptions of the anatomic landmarks that correspond with the reference numbers within the schematics of each of the individual Hayduke Breast Grids are detailed in Table 2. Reference numbers of the anatomic landmarks overlaid on human breast illustrations are depicted below for frontal (Figure 75), right profile (Figure 76), and left profile (Figure 77) breast poses. Each grid's schematic includes curly brackets labeled with the numbers 1.618 and 1.0. These labels correspond to the location of the golden ratio relationship within each grid. The location of the 1.618:1.0 ratio within a grid varies depending upon the design of the grid. Some of the grids have the 1.618:1.0 ratio in the vertical side components of the quadrilaterals within the grid, and some grids harbor the golden ratio relationship in the horizontal side components of the quadrilaterals within the grid. Several of the Hayduke Breast Grids contain a golden spiral as well as a series of golden rectangles as the core components of the grid.

Reference Number	Anatomic Description
401	base of the jugular suprasternal notch
402	medial uppermost margin of right breast where the breast tissue terminates and joins the flat parasternal area
403	medial uppermost margin of the left breast where the breast tissue terminates and joins the flat parasternal area
404	superior border of the right areola
405	superior border of the left areola
406	superior border of the right nipple
407	superior border of the left nipple
408	lateral margin of the right breast
409	lateral border of the right areola
410	center of the right nipple
411	medial border of the right areola
412	medial border of the left areola
413	center of the left nipple
414	lateral border of the left areola
415	lateral margin of the left breast
416	central inferiormost margin of the right breast
417	central inferiormost margin of the left breast
418	center of the umbilicus
419	lowermost inferior border of the right clavicle
420	superior border of the right areola
421	central base of the right nipple where the nipple base joins the areola
422	anteriormost margin of the right breast (excluding right nipple projection)
423	inferiormost central margin of the right breast
424	lowermost inferior border of the left clavicle
425	superior border of the left areola
426	central base of the left nipple where the nipple base joins the areola
427	anteriormost margin of the left breast (excluding left nipple projection)
428	inferiormost central margin of the left breast
429	anteriormost margin of the right shoulder
430	right olecranon
431	anteriormost margin of the left shoulder
432	left olecranon

Table 2. Anatomic descriptions corresponding to the reference numbers used in the Hayduke Breast Grid schematics.

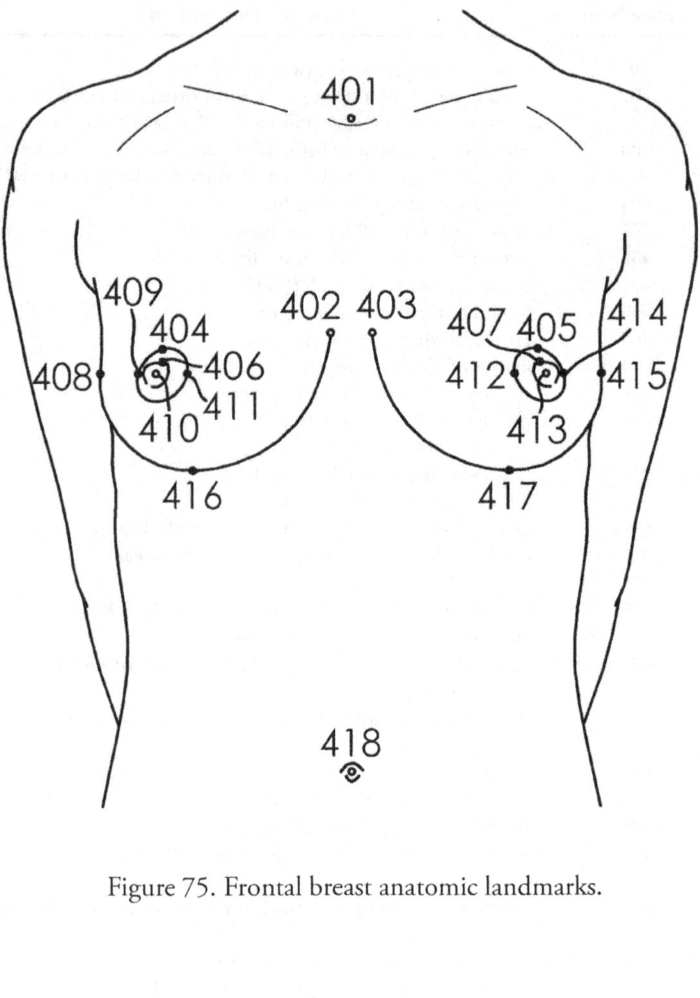

Figure 75. Frontal breast anatomic landmarks.

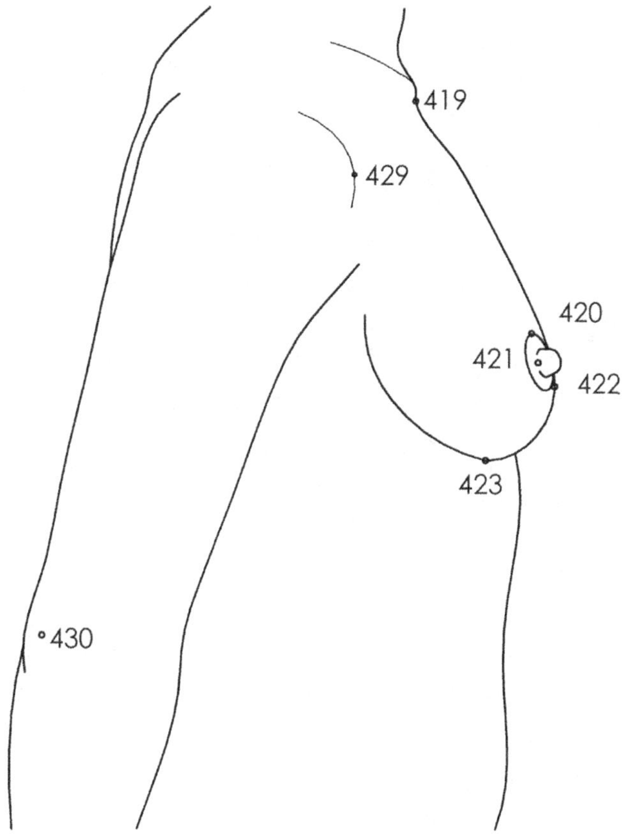

Figure 76. Right profile breast anatomic landmarks.

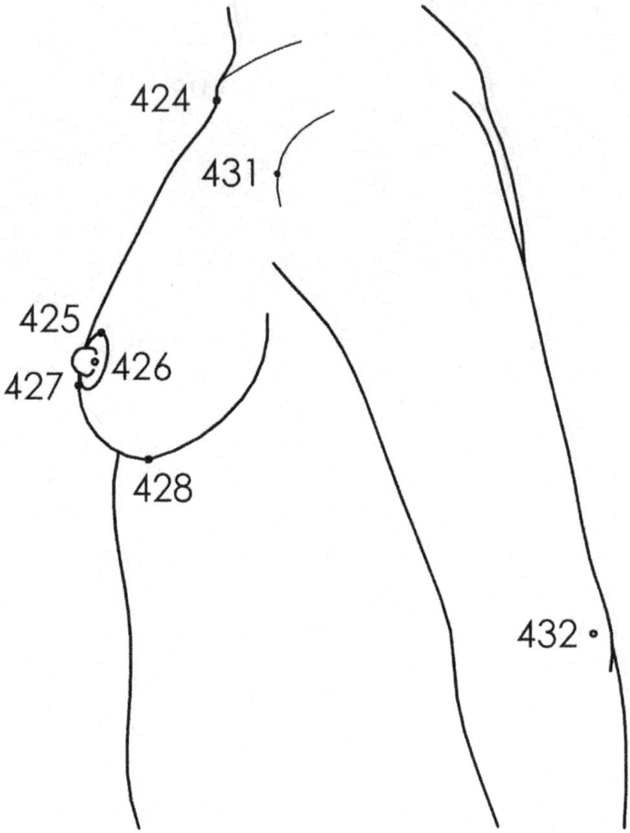

Figure 77. Left profile breast anatomic landmarks.

Hayduke Breast Grid 1 (Figure 78) is a grid with four anchor points (anatomic landmarks) that dictate the location of the three horizontal gridlines of this grid. The first anchor point is located at the base of the jugular suprasternal notch (401). This dictates the location of the uppermost horizontal gridline. The second and third anchor points are located at the superior borders of the right and left nipples (406 and 407). This dictates the location of the middle horizontal gridline. The fourth anchor point is located at the center of the umbilicus (418). This anatomic landmark dictates the location of the lowermost horizontal gridline. The grid derived from these four anchor points consists of two vertically arranged quadrilaterals. The first quadrilateral is formed between the jugular suprasternal notch (401) and the superior borders of the right and left nipples (406 and 407). The second quadrilateral is formed between the superior borders of the right and left nipples (406 and 407) and the center of the umbilicus (418). The vertical sides of these two quadrilaterals are related by the ratio 1.0:1.618.

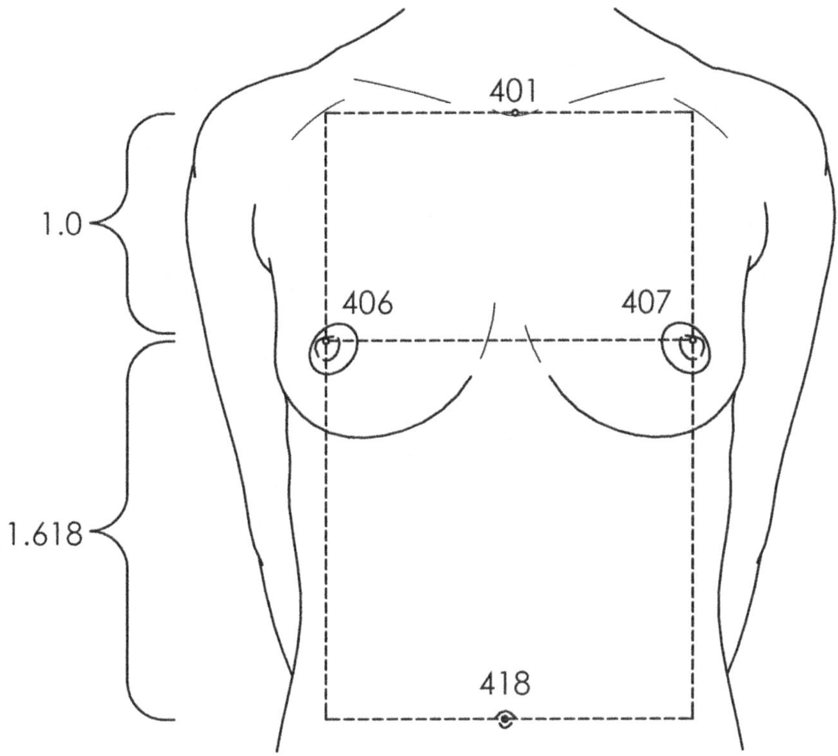

Figure 78. Hayduke Breast Grid 1.

Hayduke Breast Grid 2 (Figure 79) is a grid with three anchor points (anatomic landmarks) that dictate the location of the three horizontal gridlines of this grid. The first anchor point is located at the base of the jugular suprasternal notch (401). This anatomic landmark dictates the location of the uppermost horizontal gridline. The second anchor point is located at the superior border of the right nipple (406). This landmark dictates the location of the middle horizontal gridline. The third anchor point is located at the center of the umbilicus (418). This landmark dictates the location of the lowermost horizontal gridline. The grid derived from these three anchor points consists of two vertically arranged quadrilaterals. The first quadrilateral is formed between the jugular suprasternal notch (401) and the superior border of the right nipple (406). The second quadrilateral is formed between the superior border of the right nipple (406) and the center of the umbilicus (418). The vertical sides of these two quadrilaterals are related by the ratio 1.0:1.618.

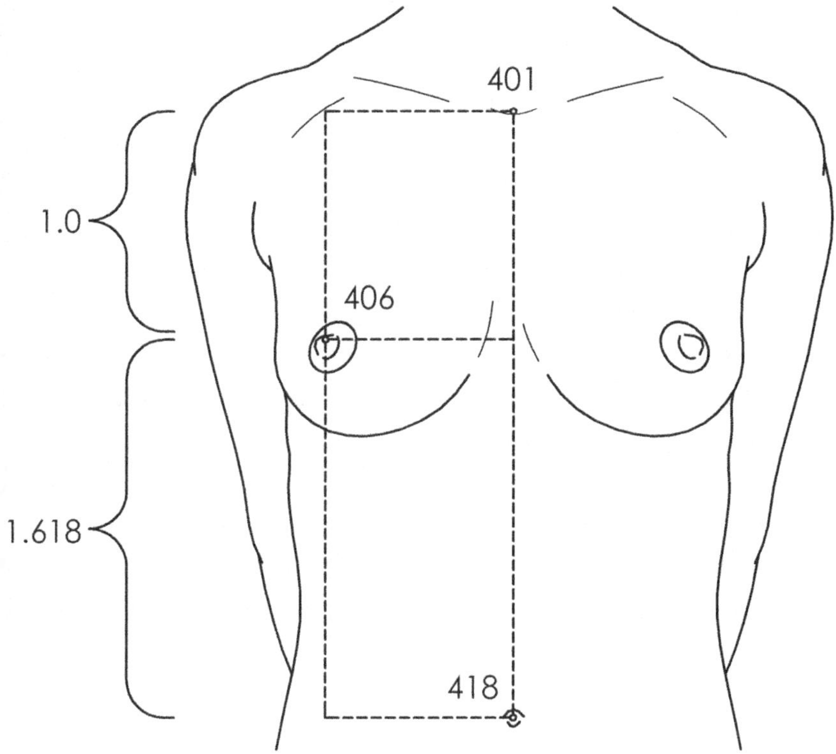

Figure 79. Hayduke Breast Grid 2.

Hayduke Breast Grid 3 (Figure 80) is a grid with three anchor points (anatomic landmarks) that dictate the location of the three horizontal gridlines of this grid. The first anchor point is located at the base of the jugular suprasternal notch (401). This dictates the location of the uppermost horizontal gridline. The second anchor point is located at the superior border of the left nipple (407). This dictates the location of the middle horizontal gridline. The third anchor point is located at the center of the umbilicus (418). This dictates the location of the lowermost horizontal gridline. The grid derived from these three anchor points consists of two vertically arranged quadrilaterals. The first quadrilateral is formed between the jugular suprasternal notch (401) and the superior border of the left nipple (407). The second quadrilateral is formed between the superior border of the left nipple (407) and the center of the umbilicus (418). The vertical sides of these two quadrilaterals are related by the ratio 1.0:1.618.

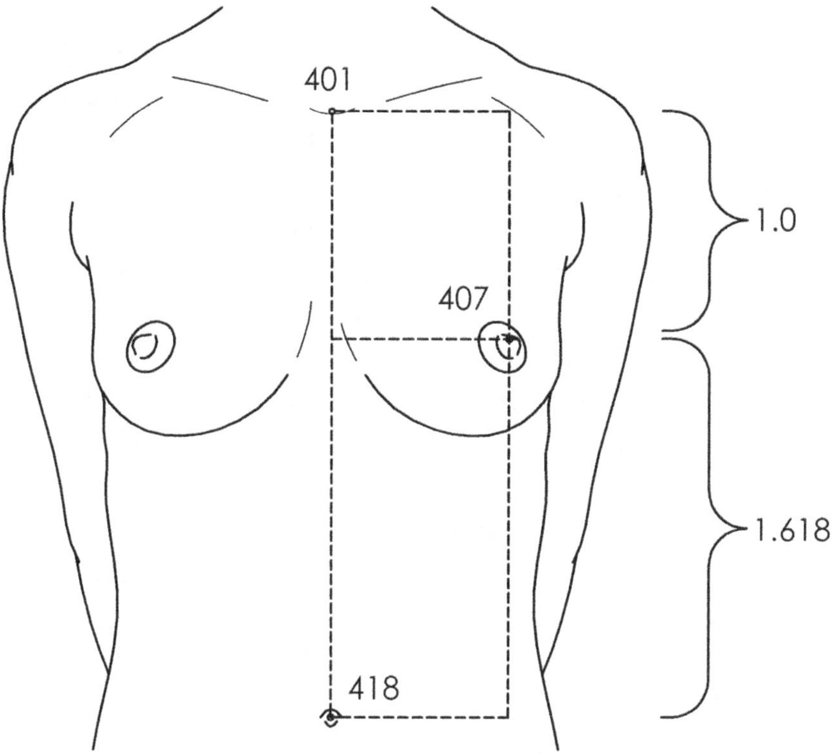

Figure 80. Hayduke Breast Grid 3.

Hayduke Breast Grid 4 (Figure 81) is a grid with five anchor points (anatomic landmarks) that dictate the location of the three horizontal gridlines of this grid. The first anchor point is located at the base of the jugular suprasternal notch (401). This anchor point dictates the location of the uppermost horizontal gridline. The second and third anchor points are located at the superior borders of the right and left areolas (404 and 405). These anchor points dictate the location of the middle horizontal gridline. The fourth and fifth anchor points are located at the inferior margins of the right and left breasts (416 and 417). These points dictate the location of the lowermost horizontal gridline. Two vertically arranged quadrilaterals of this grid are derived from these anchor points. In this overlay, the first quadrilateral is formed between the jugular suprasternal notch (401) and the superior borders of the right and left areolas (404 and 405). The second quadrilateral is formed between the superior border of the right and left areolas (404 and 405) and the inferior margins of the right and left breasts (416 and 417). The vertical sides of these two quadrilaterals are related by the ratio 1.618:1.0.

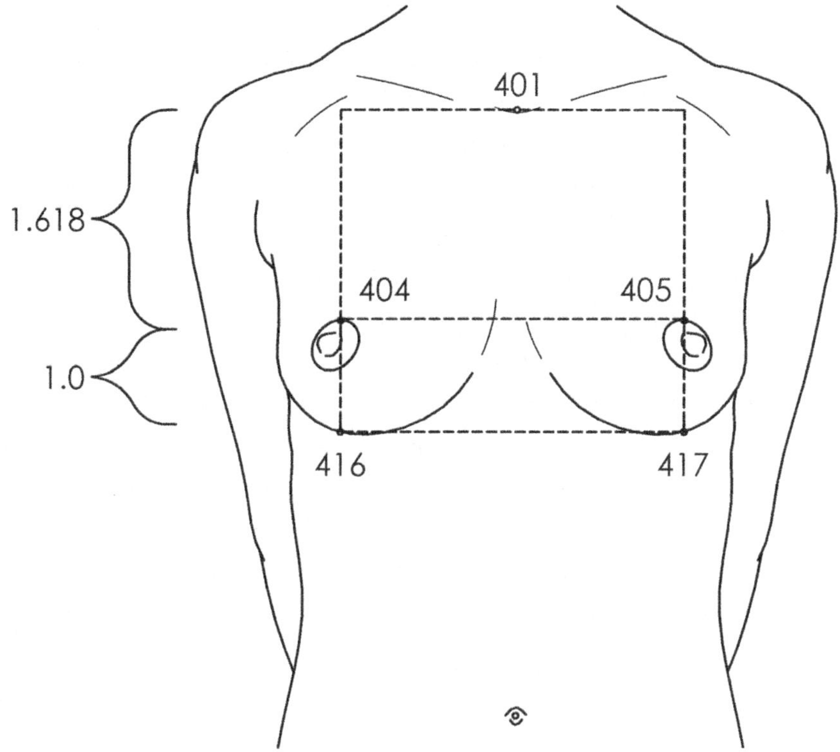

Figure 81. Hayduke Breast Grid 4.

Hayduke Breast Grid 5 (Figure 82) is a grid with three anchor points (anatomic landmarks) that dictate the location of the three horizontal gridlines of this grid. The first anchor point is located at the base of the jugular suprasternal notch (401). This point dictates the location of the uppermost horizontal gridline. The second anchor point is located at the superior margin of the right areola (404). This point dictates the location of the middle horizontal gridline. The third anchor point is located at the inferior margin of the right breast (416). This point dictates the location of the lowermost horizontal gridline. Two vertically arranged quadrilaterals are formed. In this overlay, the first quadrilateral is formed between the jugular suprasternal notch (401) and the superior border of the right areola (404). The second quadrilateral is formed between the superior border of the right areola (404) and the inferior margin of the right breast (416). The vertical sides of these two quadrilaterals are related by the ratio 1.618:1.0.

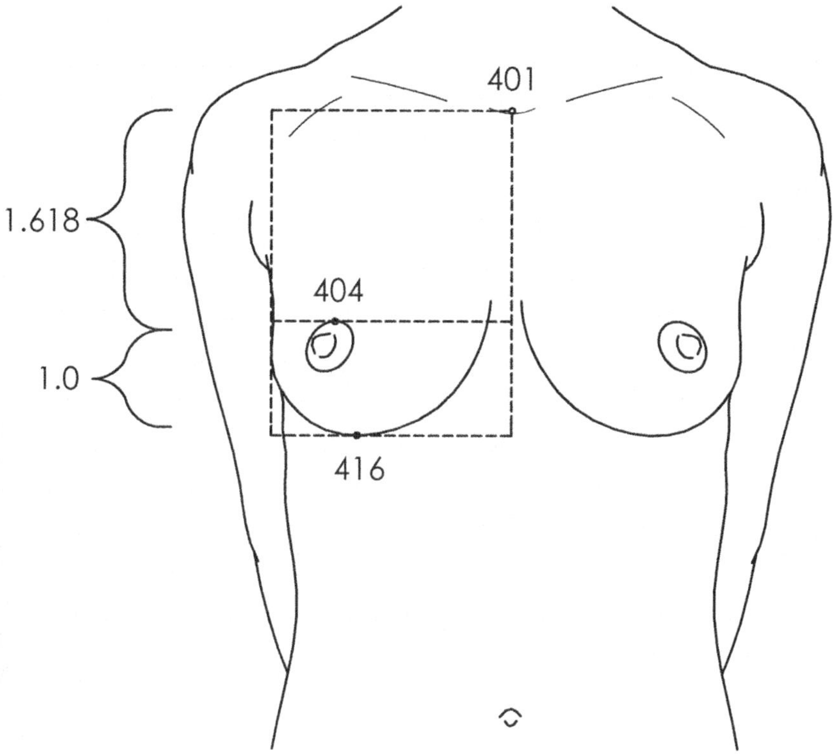

Figure 82. Hayduke Breast Grid 5.

Hayduke Breast Grid 6 (Figure 83) is a grid with three anchor points (anatomic landmarks) that dictate the location of the three horizontal gridlines of this grid. The first anchor point is located at the base of the jugular suprasternal notch (401). This point dictates the location of the uppermost horizontal gridline. The second anchor point is located at the superior margin of the left areola (405). This point dictates the location of the middle horizontal gridline. The third anchor point is located at the inferior margin of the right breast (417). This point dictates the location of the lowermost horizontal gridline. These gridlines form two vertically arranged quadrilaterals. In this overlay, the first quadrilateral is formed between the jugular suprasternal notch (401) and the superior border of the left areola (405). The second quadrilateral is formed between the superior border of the left areola (405) and the inferior margin of the left breast (417). The vertical sides of these two quadrilaterals are related by the ratio 1.618:1.0.

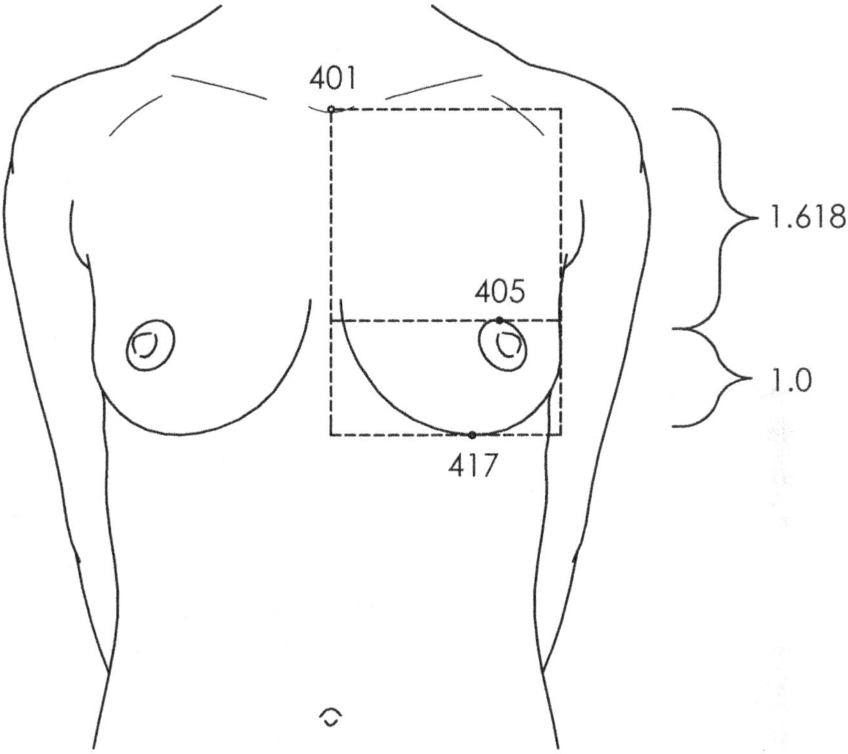

Figure 83. Hayduke Breast Grid 6.

Hayduke Breast Grid 7 (Figure 84) is a right-sided breast grid based on a series of golden rectangles with a golden spiral located within this series of golden rectangles. A golden rectangle is a four-sided figure having four right angles whose long-to-short side lengths can be reduced to the golden ratio (1.618:1.0). The ratio of the long side to short side of a golden rectangle is 1.618:1.0. When a square shape is removed from the outer (largest) golden rectangle, the remainder forms another golden rectangle, that is, one having the same aspect ratio as the original golden rectangle but with a smaller overall size. Hayduke Breast Grid 7 depicts squares being removed sequentially starting from the uppermost part of the outer (largest) vertically oriented golden rectangle and proceeding in a clockwise sequence. This process is repeated a total of six times. This creates the gridline layout of the golden rectangles within Hayduke Breast Grid 7. The golden spiral is a logarithmic spiral whose growth factor is 1.618 and follows the series of golden rectangles within Hayduke Breast Grid 7. The golden spiral's growth causes its edge to move farther from its origin by a factor of 1.618 for every counterclockwise quarter turn of growth. The golden spiral within Hayduke Breast Grid 7 originates in the smallest square's superolateral corner, spirals counterclockwise, and terminates in the superolateral corner of the grid's largest square. Three anchor points determine both the location of three of the grid's outer golden rectangle sides as well as the overall size of the outer (largest) golden rectangle of Hayduke Breast Grid 7. The medial (inner) vertical long side of the outer golden rectangle is determined by an anchor point defined by the medialmost (inner) margin of the right breast (402). The lowermost side of the outer golden rectangle is determined by an anchor point defined by the central, inferiormost margin of the right breast (416). The lateral (outer) vertical long side of the outer golden rectangle is determined by an anchor point defined by the lateralmost (outer) margin of the right breast (408). Overlay placement of Hayduke Breast Grid 7 based on these three anchor points on a frontal, right breast image allows evaluation of right-sided breast anatomy that includes evaluation of the lower pole curvature of the right breast as it relates to the golden spiral as well as the location of the medial border of the right areola (411) and the location of the right nipple (410).

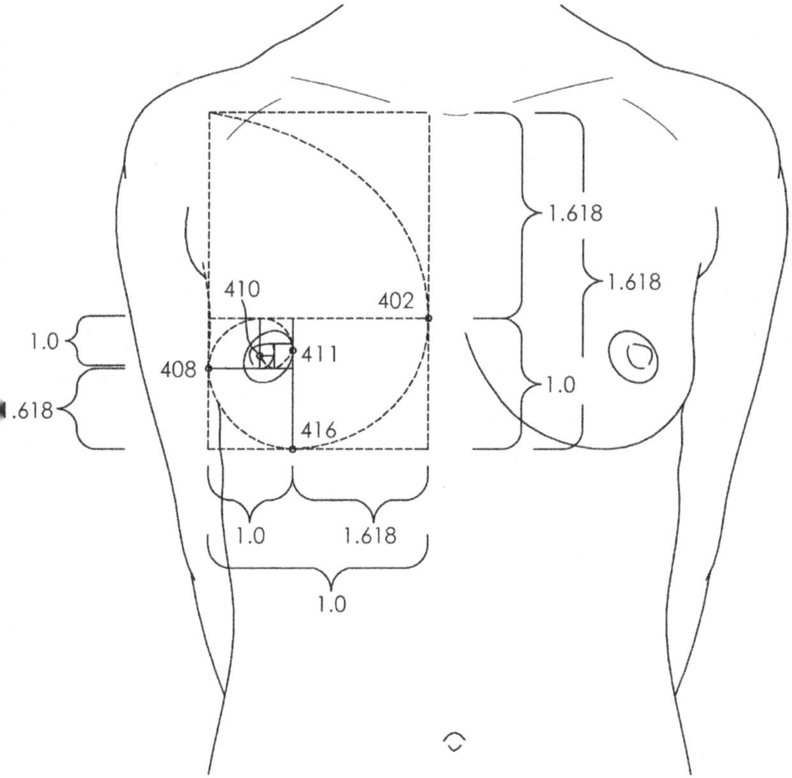

Figure 84. Hayduke Breast Grid 7.

Hayduke Breast Grid 8 (Figure 85) is a left-sided breast grid based on a series of golden rectangles with a golden spiral located within this series of golden rectangles. A golden rectangle is a four-sided figure having four right angles whose long-to-short side lengths can be reduced to the golden ratio (1.618:1.0). The ratio of the long side to short side of a golden rectangle is 1.618:1.0. When a square shape is removed from the outer (largest) golden rectangle, the remainder forms another golden rectangle, that is, one having the same aspect ratio as the original golden rectangle but with a smaller overall size. Hayduke Breast Grid 8 depicts squares being removed sequentially starting from the uppermost part of the outer (largest) vertically oriented golden rectangle and proceeding in a counterclockwise sequence. This process is repeated a total of six times. This creates the gridline layout of the golden rectangles within Hayduke Breast Grid 8. The golden spiral is a logarithmic spiral whose growth factor is 1.618 and follows the series of golden rectangles within Hayduke Breast Grid 8. The golden spiral's growth causes its edge to move farther from its origin by a factor of 1.618 for every clockwise quarter turn of growth. The golden spiral within Hayduke Breast Grid 8 originates in the smallest square's superolateral corner, spirals clockwise, and terminates in the superolateral corner of the grid's largest square. Three anchor points determine both the location of three of the grid's outer golden rectangle sides as well as the overall size of the outer (largest) golden rectangle of Hayduke Breast Grid 8. The medial (inner) vertical long side of the outer golden rectangle is determined by an anchor point defined by the medialmost (inner) margin of the left breast (403). The lowermost side of the outer golden rectangle is determined by an anchor point defined by the central inferiormost margin of the left breast (417). The lateral (outer) vertical long side of the outer golden rectangle is determined by an anchor point defined by the lateralmost (outer) margin of the left breast (415). Overlay placement of Hayduke Breast Grid 8 based on these three anchor points on a frontal left breast image allows evaluation of left sided breast anatomy that includes evaluation of the lower pole curvature of the left breast as it relates to the golden spiral as well as the location of the medial border of the left areola (412) and the location of the left nipple (413).

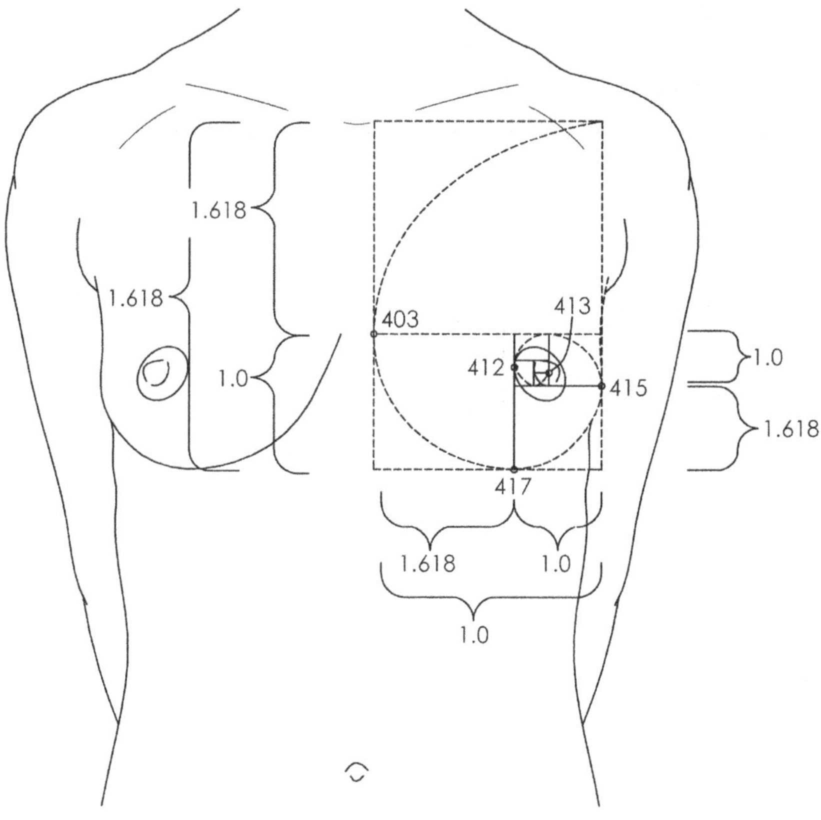

Figure 85. Hayduke Breast Grid 8.

Hayduke Breast Grid 9 (Figure 86) is a grid with three anchor points (anatomic landmarks) that dictate the location of the three vertical gridlines of this grid. The first anchor point is the medial-most (inner) margin of the right breast (402). The second anchor point is located at the medial (inner) border of the right areola (411). The third anchor point is located at the lateralmost (outer) margin of the right breast (408). Two horizontally arranged quadrilaterals are formed. In this overlay, the first quadrilateral is formed between the medial margin of the right breast (402) and the medial border of the right areola (411). The second quadrilateral is formed between the medial border of the right areola (411) and the lateral-most margin of the right breast (408). The horizontal sides of these two quadrilaterals are related by the ratio 1.618:1.0.

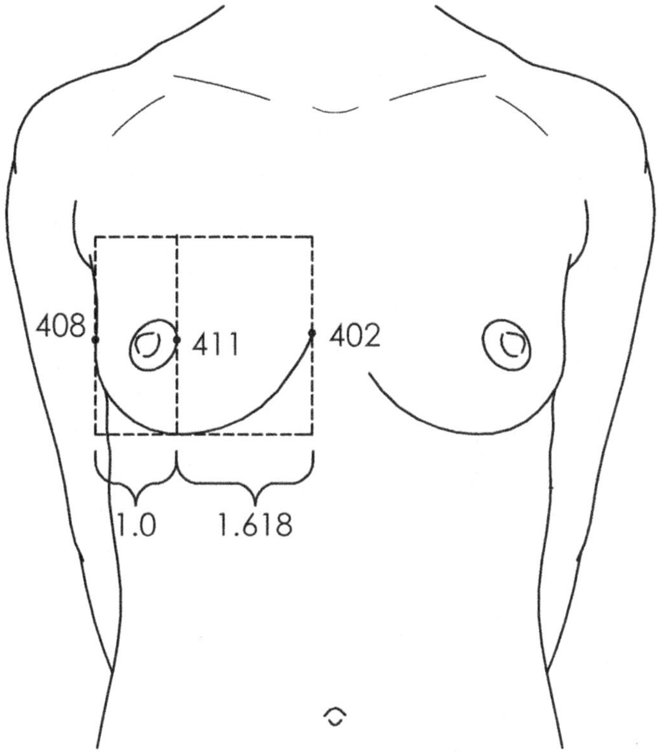

Figure 86. Hayduke Breast Grid 9.

Hayduke Breast Grid 10 (Figure 87) is a grid with three anchor points (anatomic landmarks) that dictate the location of the three vertical gridlines of this grid. The first anchor point is located at the medialmost (inner) margin of the left breast (403). The second anchor point is located at the medial (inner) border of the left areola (412). The third anchor point is located at the lateralmost (outer) margin of the left breast (415). Two horizontally arranged quadrilaterals are formed. In this overlay, the first quadrilateral is formed between the medial margin of the left breast (403) and the medial border of the left areola (412). The second quadrilateral is formed between the medial border of the left areola (412) and the lateralmost margin of the left breast (415). The horizontal sides of these two quadrilaterals are related by the ratio 1.618:1.0.

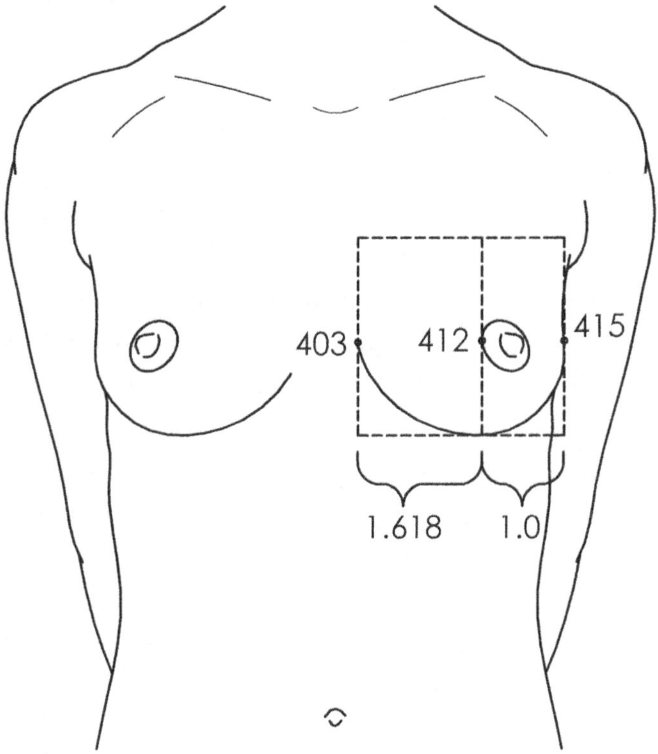

Figure 87. Hayduke Breast Grid 10.

Hayduke Breast Grid 11 (Figure 88) is a grid composed of three horizontally arranged quadrilaterals. The horizontal sides of the outer two quadrilaterals of this grid are related to the horizontal side of the central quadrilateral by the ratio 1.618:1.0. The overall size (width) of Hayduke Breast Grid 11 is first set using specific anchor points (anatomic landmarks). The grid, with its width set by these anchor points, is then hovered over the right areola to determine if the areolar diameter (distance between points 409 and 411) fits within the central quadrilateral of Hayduke Breast Grid 11. To set the overall width of this grid, two anchor points (anatomic landmarks) are used to determine the location of the two outermost vertical gridlines of this grid. The first anchor point is the medialmost (inner) margin of the right breast. This anatomic landmark is depicted as point 402 in Figure 75. This sets the inner vertical gridline location for setting the overall grid size. The second anchor point is the lateralmost (outer) margin of the right breast. This anatomic landmark is depicted as point 408 in Figure 75. This sets the outermost vertical gridline location for setting the overall grid size of Hayduke Breast Grid 11. The two vertical gridlines created by these two anchor points set the overall width of Hayduke Breast Grid 11 while maintaining the horizontal side relationships of 1.618:1.0 of the three quadrilaterals. While maintaining the already set grid width (size), this overlay grid is now hovered over the right areola to determine if the diameter of the right areola (distance between points 409 and 411) fits the central quadrilateral of Hayduke Breast Grid 11. This relates the areolar diameter to the total frontal width of the entire breast based on golden ratio relationships.

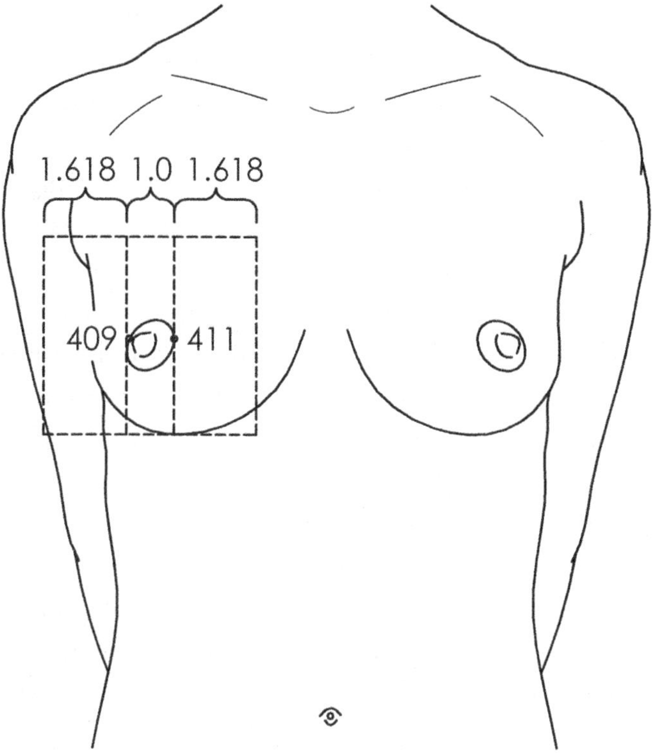

Figure 88. Hayduke Breast Grid 11.

Hayduke Breast Grid 12 (Figure 89) is a grid composed of three horizontally arranged quadrilaterals. The horizontal sides of the outer two quadrilaterals of this grid are related to the horizontal side of the central quadrilateral by the ratio 1.618:1.0. The overall size (width) of Hayduke Breast Grid 12 is first set using specific anchor points (anatomic landmarks). The grid, with its width set by these anchor points, is then hovered over the left areola to determine if the areolar diameter (distance between points 412 and 414) fits within the central quadrilateral of Hayduke Breast Grid 12. To set the overall width of this grid, two anchor points (anatomic landmarks) are used to determine the location of the two outermost vertical gridlines of this grid. The first anchor point is the medialmost (inner) margin of the left breast. This anatomic landmark point is depicted as point 403 in Figure 75. This sets the inner vertical gridline location for setting the overall grid size. The second anchor point is the lateralmost (outer) margin of the left breast. This anatomic landmark is depicted as point 415 in Figure 75. This sets the outermost vertical gridline location for setting the overall grid size. The two vertical gridlines created by these two anchor points set the overall width (size) of Hayduke Breast Grid 12 while maintaining the horizontal side relationships of 1.618:1.0 of the three quadrilaterals (Figure 89). While maintaining the already set grid width (size), this overlay grid is now hovered over the left areola to determine if the diameter of the left areola (distance between points 412 and 414) fits the central quadrilateral of Hayduke Breast Grid 12. This relates the areolar diameter to the total frontal width of the entire breast based upon golden ratio relationships.

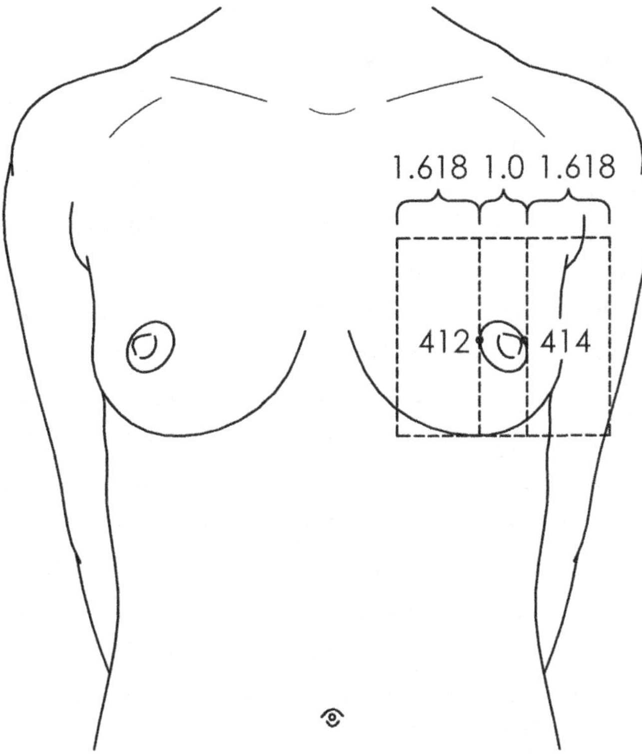

Figure 89. Hayduke Breast Grid 12.

Hayduke Breast Grid 13 (Figure 90) is a right-profile grid with three anchor points (anatomic landmarks) that dictate the location of the three horizontal gridlines of this grid. The first anchor point is located at the inferior (lowermost) border of the clavicle at the anterior profile skin margin (419). This point dictates the location of the uppermost horizontal gridline. The second anchor point is located at the superior border of the right areola (420). This point dictates the location of the middle horizontal gridline. The third anchor point is located at the lowermost inferior margin of the right breast (423). This point dictates the location of the lowermost horizontal gridline. The grid derived from these three anchor points consists of two vertically arranged quadrilaterals. The first quadrilateral is formed between the inferior border of the clavicle (419) and the superior border of the areola (420). The second quadrilateral is formed between the superior border of the areola (420) and the inferior margin of the right breast (423). The vertical side of the first quadrilateral is related to the vertical side of the second quadrilateral by the ratio 1.618:1.0.

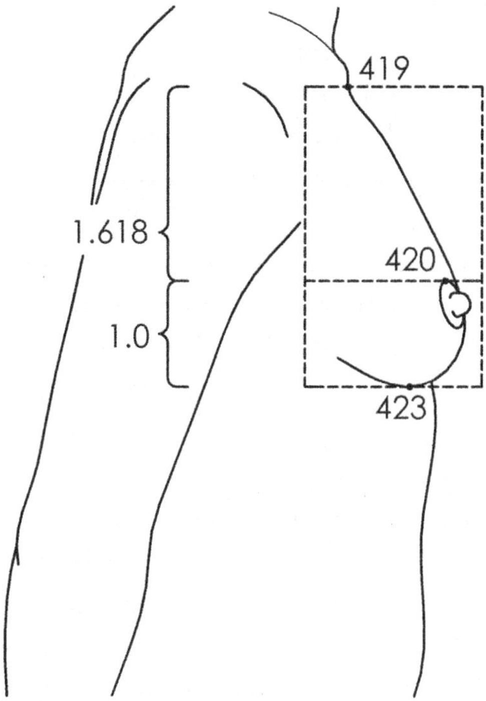

Figure 90. Hayduke Breast Grid 13.

Hayduke Breast Grid 14 (Figure 91) is a left-profile breast grid with three anchor points (anatomic landmarks) that dictate the location of the three horizontal gridlines of this grid. The first anchor point is located at the inferior (lowermost) border of the clavicle at the anterior profile skin margin (424). This point dictates the location of the uppermost horizontal gridline. The second anchor point is located at the superior border of the left areola (425). This point dictates the location of the middle horizontal gridline. The third anchor point is located at the lowermost inferior margin of the left breast (428). This point dictates the location of the lowermost horizontal gridline. The grid derived from these three anchor points consists of two vertically arranged quadrilaterals. The first quadrilateral is formed between the inferior border of the clavicle (424) and the superior border of the areola (425). The second quadrilateral is formed between the superior border of the areola (425) and the inferior margin of the left breast (428). The vertical side of the first quadrilateral is related to the vertical side of the second quadrilateral by the ratio 1.618:1.0.

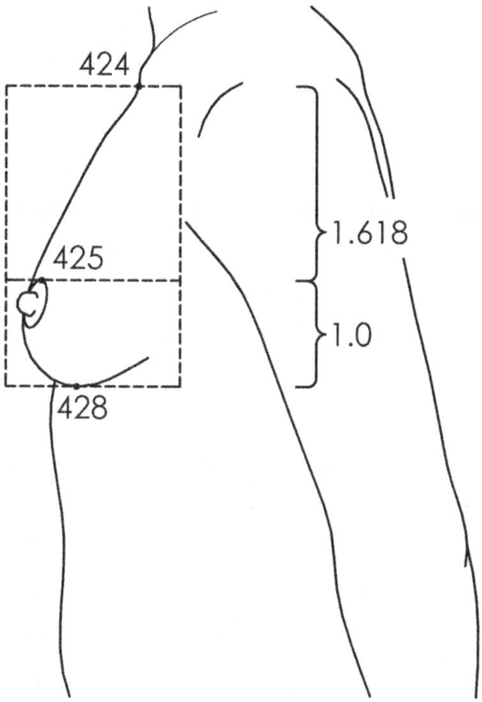

Figure 91. Hayduke Breast Grid 14.

Hayduke Breast Grid 15 (Figure 92) is a right-profile grid based on a series of golden rectangles with a golden spiral located within this series of golden rectangles. A golden rectangle is a four-sided figure having four right angles whose long-to-short side lengths can be reduced to the golden ratio (1.618:1.0). The ratio of the long side to short side of a golden rectangle is 1.618:1.0. When a square shape is removed from the outer (largest) golden rectangle, the remainder forms another golden rectangle, that is, one having the same aspect ratio as the original golden rectangle but with a smaller overall size. Sequential square removal is started from the uppermost part of the outer (largest) vertically oriented golden rectangle and is repeated three times total starting from the outer (largest) golden rectangle in a counterclockwise sequence to create the gridlines of Hayduke Breast Grid 15. The golden spiral is a logarithmic spiral having a growth factor of 1.618 and follows this series of golden rectangles within Hayduke Breast Grid 15. The golden spiral's growth causes its edge to move farther from its origin by a factor of 1.618 for every clockwise quarter turn of growth. The golden spiral originates from the upper anterior corner of the smallest square within Hayduke Breast Grid 15 and its tail terminates in the upper anterior-most corner of the largest golden rectangle away from a subject's image. Two anchor points dictate both the location of the upper and lower horizontal short side positions of the outer golden rectangle of this grid as well as the overall size of the outer (largest) golden rectangle of this grid. The first anchor point is located at the lowermost inferior border of the clavicle at the anterior profile skin margin (419). This dictates the location of the uppermost horizontal short side of the rectangle. The second anchor point is located at the lowermost inferior margin of the right breast (423). This dictates the location of the lowermost horizontal short side of the rectangle. With the overall grid size set by these two anchor points, the grid is then hovered over the right breast to set the golden spiral over the central, inferiormost anchor point of the lower right breast margin. The part of the golden spiral that's lined up with the central, inferiormost anchor point of the right breast is the posteriorly directed takeoff point of the golden spiral curve as it leaves the lowermost outer (largest) rectangle short side. Overlay placement of Hayduke Breast Grid 15 based on these anchor points of a right breast profile image allows evaluation of right sided breast anatomy that includes evaluation of right breast anterior projection, overall breast size, and lower breast curvature as it relates to the golden spiral within Hayduke Breast Grid 15.

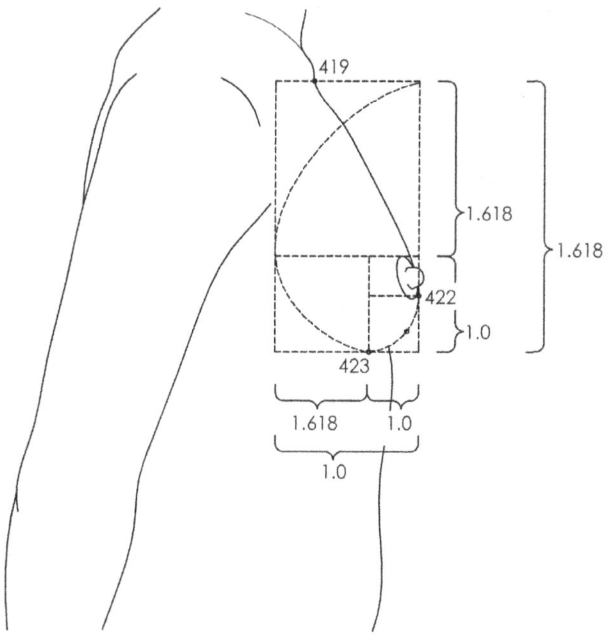

Figure 92. Hayduke Breast Grid 15.

Hayduke Breast Grid 16 (Figure 93) is a left-profile grid based on a series of golden rectangles with a golden spiral located within this series of golden rectangles. A golden rectangle is a four-sided figure having four right angles whose long-to-short side lengths can be reduced to the golden ratio (1.618:1.0). The ratio of the long side to short side of the golden rectangle is 1.618:1.0. When a square shape is removed from the outer (largest) golden rectangle, the remainder forms another golden rectangle, that is, one having the same aspect ratio as the original golden rectangle but with a smaller overall size. Sequential square removal is started from the uppermost part of the outer (largest) vertically oriented golden rectangle and is repeated three times total starting from the outer (largest) golden rectangle in a clockwise sequence to create the gridlines of Hayduke Breast Grid 16. The golden spiral is a logarithmic spiral having a growth factor of 1.618 and follows this series of golden rectangles within this grid. The golden spiral's growth causes its edge to move farther from its origin by a factor of 1.618 for every counterclockwise quarter turn of growth. The golden spiral originates from the upper anterior corner of the smallest square within this grid and its tail terminates in the upper anterior-most corner of the largest golden rectangle away from the subject's image. Two anchor points dictate both the location of the upper and lower horizontal short side positions of the outer (largest) golden rectangle for this grid as well as the overall size of the outer (largest) golden rectangle of Hayduke Breast Grid 16. The first anchor point is located at the lowermost inferior border of the clavicle at the anterior profile skin margin (424). This dictates the location of the uppermost horizontal short side of the outer (largest) rectangle. The second anchor point is located at the lowermost inferior margin of the right breast (428). This dictates the location of the lowermost horizontal short side of the outer (largest) rectangle. With the overall grid size set by these two anchor points, the grid is then hovered over the left breast to set the golden spiral over the central, inferiormost anchor point (428) of the lower left breast margin. The part of the golden spiral that's lined up with the central, inferiormost anchor point of the left breast is the posteriorly directed takeoff point of the golden spiral curve as it leaves the lowermost outer rectangle short side. Overlay placement of Hayduke Breast Grid 16 based on these anchor points of a left breast profile image allows evaluation of left-sided breast anatomy. This includes evaluation of left-sided breast anterior projection from the profile view, overall breast size, and lower breast curvature as it relates to the golden spiral within Hayduke Breast Grid 16.

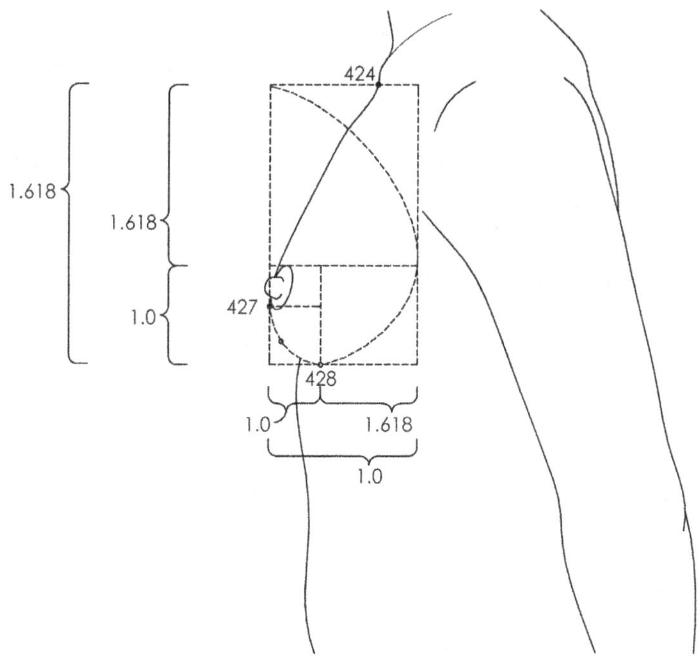

Figure 93. Hayduke Breast Grid 16.

Hayduke Breast Grid 17 (Figure 94) is a right-profile breast grid based on a series of golden rectangles. A golden rectangle is a four-sided figure having four right angles whose long-to-short side lengths can be reduced to the golden ratio (1.618:1.0). The ratio of the long side to short side of the golden rectangle is 1.618:1.0. When a square shape is removed from the outer (largest) golden rectangle, the remainder is another golden rectangle that is the same aspect ratio but smaller in overall size. Sequential square removal is started from the uppermost part of the outer (largest) vertically oriented golden rectangle and repeated three times starting from the outer (largest) golden rectangle in a counterclockwise sequence to create the multiple golden rectangle layout of Hayduke Breast Grid 17. This creates a total of four golden rectangles. Two anchor points determine the location of upper and lower horizontal short side positions of the outer (largest) golden rectangle of Hayduke Breast Grid 17 as well as the overall size of the outer (largest) golden rectangle of Hayduke Breast Grid 17. The first anchor point is located at the lowermost inferior border of the clavicle at the anterior profile skin margin (419). This point dictates the location of the uppermost horizontal short side of the outer (largest) rectangle. The second anchor point is located at the lowermost inferior margin of the right breast (423). This dictates the location of the lowermost horizontal short side of the outer (largest) rectangle. With the overall grid size set by these two anchor points, the grid is then hovered over the right breast to set the anterior vertical side of the outer golden rectangle to the most anterior projecting part of the right breast profile that doesn't include the projection of the nipple as part of the profile (422). Overlay placement of Hayduke Breast Grid 17, based on these anchor points of a right breast profile image, allows evaluation of right-sided breast anatomy. This includes evaluation of the right breast nipple base position (indicated by the small circle in Figure 94) within the smallest horizontally oriented golden rectangle inside Hayduke Breast Grid 17.

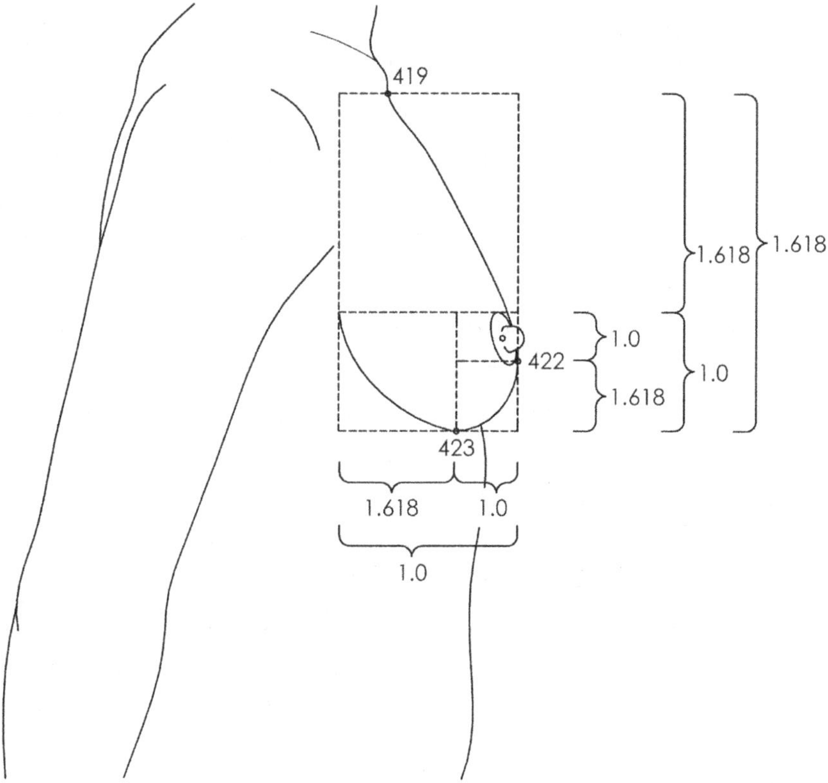

Figure 94. Hayduke Breast Grid 17.

Hayduke Breast Grid 18 (Figure 95) is a left-profile grid based on a series of golden rectangles. A golden rectangle is a four-sided figure having four right angles whose long-to-short side lengths can be reduced to the golden ratio (1.618:1.0). The ratio of the long side to short side of the golden rectangle is 1.618:1.0. When a square shape is removed from the outer (largest) golden rectangle, the remainder is another golden rectangle that has the same aspect ratio but is smaller in overall size. Sequential square removal is started from the uppermost part of the outer (largest) vertically oriented golden rectangle and is repeated three times total starting from the outer (largest) golden rectangle in a clockwise sequence to create the multiple golden rectangle layout of Hayduke Breast Grid 18. This creates a total of four golden rectangles. Two anchor points dictate both the location of upper and lower horizontal short side positions of the outer (largest) golden rectangle as well as the overall size of the outer (largest) golden rectangle of Hayduke Breast Grid 18. The first anchor point is located at the lowermost inferior border of the clavicle at the anterior profile skin margin (424). This dictates the location of the uppermost horizontal short side of the outer (largest) rectangle. The second anchor point is located at the lowermost inferior margin of the right breast (428). This dictates the location of the lowermost horizontal short side of the outer (largest) rectangle. With the overall grid size set by these two anchor points, the grid is then hovered over the left breast to set the anterior vertical side of the outer golden rectangle to the most anterior projecting part of the left breast profile that doesn't include the projection of the nipple off of the breast as part of the profile (427). Overlay placement of Hayduke Breast Grid 17 based on these anchor points of a left breast profile image allows evaluation of left-sided breast anatomy. This includes evaluation of the left breast nipple base position (indicated by the small circle in Figure 95) within the smallest horizontally oriented golden rectangle inside Hayduke Breast Grid 18.

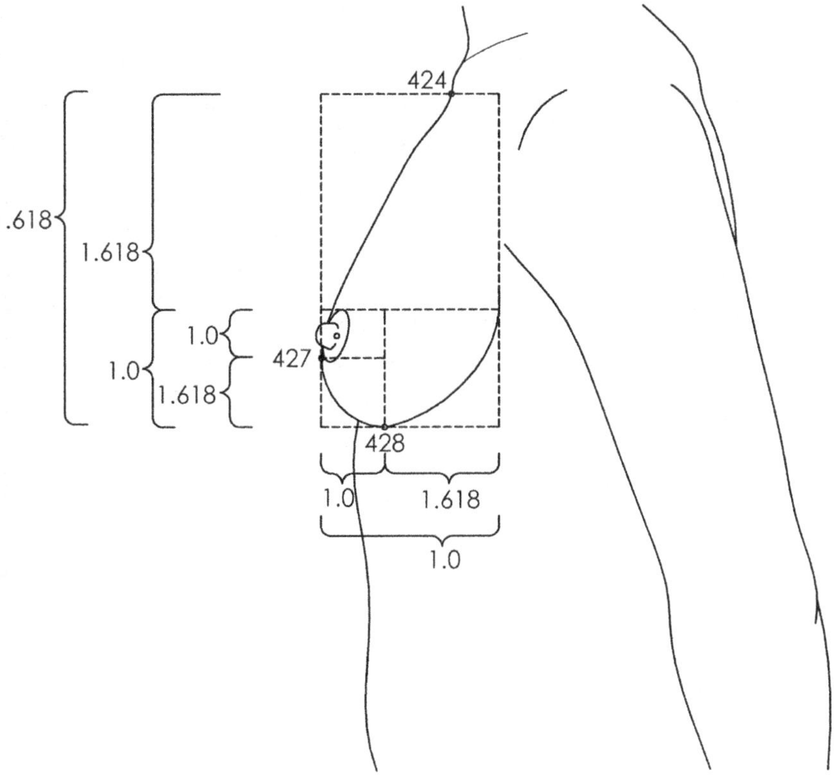

Figure 95. Hayduke Breast Grid 18.

Hayduke Breast Grid 19 (Figure 96) is a grid with three anchor points that dictate the location of the three horizontal gridlines of this grid. The first anchor point is located at the anteriormost margin of the right shoulder (429). This dictates the position of the upper horizontal gridline. The second anchor point is located at the central base of the right nipple where the nipple base joins the areola (421). This dictates the position of the middle horizontal gridline. The third anchor point is located at the right olecranon (430). This dictates the location of the lowermost horizontal gridline. These three anchor points form two vertically arranged quadrilaterals. The first quadrilateral is formed between the anteriormost margin of the right shoulder (429) and the central base of the right nipple where the nipple base joins the areola (421). The second quadrilateral is formed between the central base of the right nipple, where the nipple base joins the areola (421), and the right olecranon (430). The vertical side of the first quadrilateral is related to the vertical side of the second quadrilateral by the ratio 1.0:1.618.

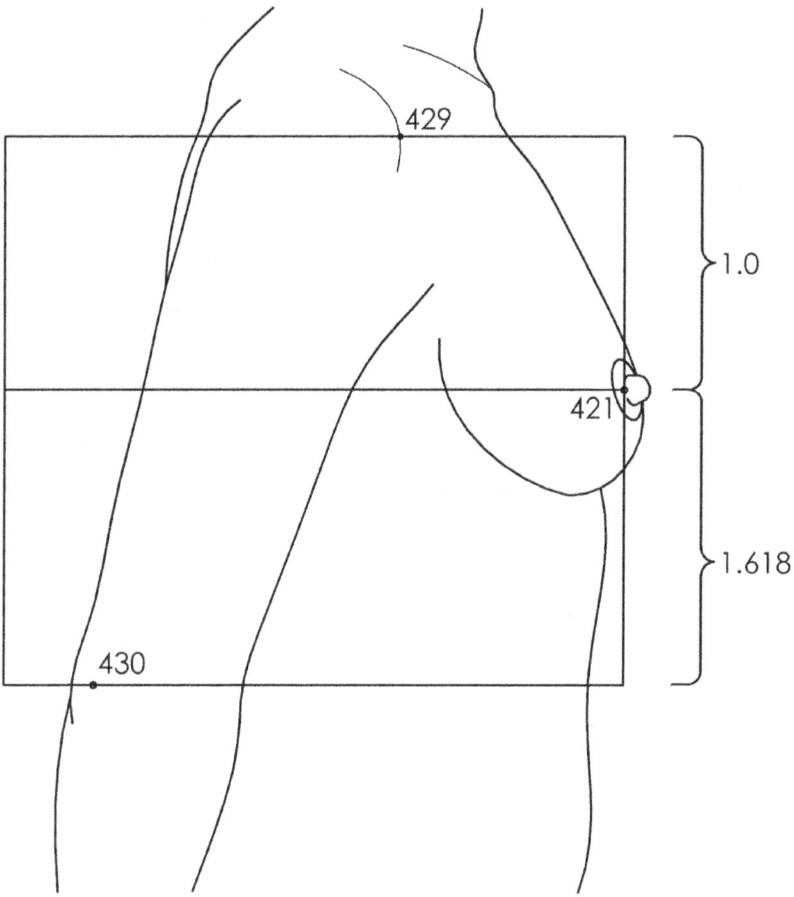

Figure 96. Hayduke Breast Grid 19.

Hayduke Breast Grid 20 (Figure 97) is a grid with three anchor points (anatomic landmarks) that dictate the location of the three horizontal gridlines of this grid. The first anchor point is located at the anteriormost margin of the left shoulder (431). This point dictates the location of the upper horizontal gridline. The second anchor point is located at the central base of the left nipple where the nipple base joins the areola (426). This point dictates the location of the middle horizontal gridline. The third anchor point is located at the left olecranon (432). This point dictates the location of the lowermost horizontal gridline. The grid derived from these three anchor points consists of two vertically arranged quadrilaterals. The first quadrilateral is formed between the anteriormost margin of the left shoulder (431) and the central base of the left nipple where the nipple base joins the areola (426). The second quadrilateral is formed between the central base of the left nipple, where the nipple base joins the areola (426), and the left olecranon (432). The vertical side of the first quadrilateral is related to the vertical side of the second quadrilateral by the ratio 1.0:1.618.

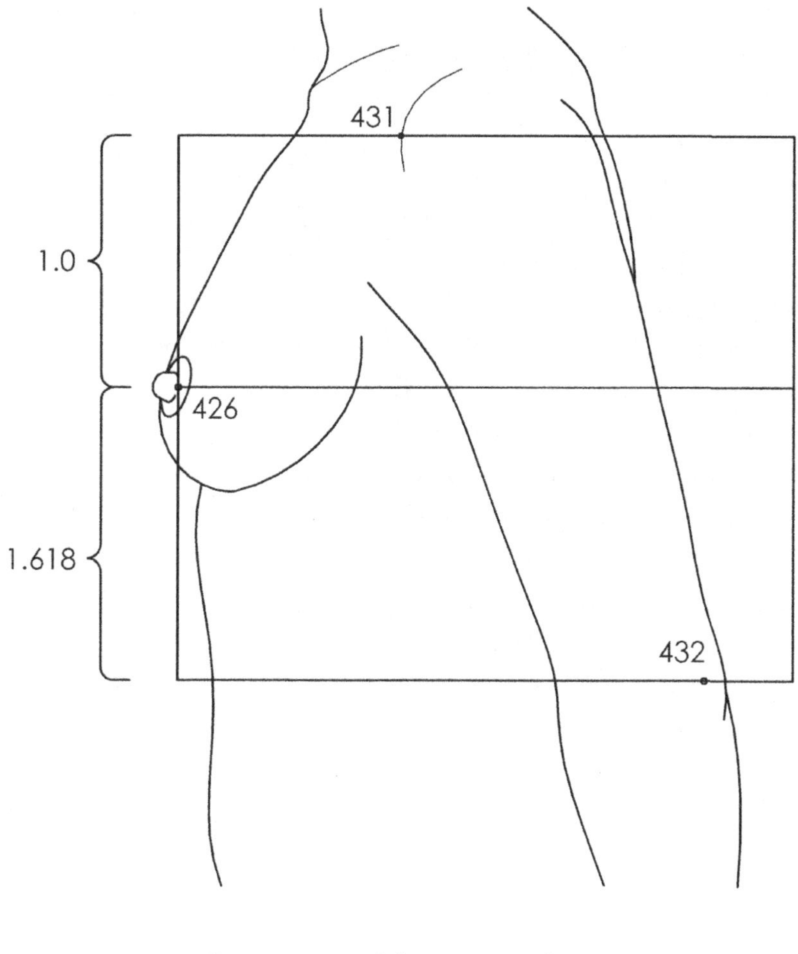

Figure 97. Hayduke Breast Grid 20.

Hayduke Breast Grid 21 (Figure 98) is a grid with three anchor points (anatomic landmarks) that dictate the location of the three horizontal gridlines of this grid. The first anchor point is located at the lowermost inferior border of the right clavicle (419). This point dictates the location of the upper horizontal gridline. The second anchor point is located at the inferior, lowermost, central margin of the right breast (423). This point dictates the position of the middle horizontal gridline. The third anchor point is located at the right olecranon (430). This point dictates the position of the lowermost horizontal gridline. The grid derived from these three anchor points consists of two vertically arranged quadrilaterals. The first quadrilateral is formed between the lowermost inferior border of the right clavicle (419) and the inferior, lowermost, central margin of the right breast (423). The second quadrilateral is formed between the inferior, lowermost, central margin of the right breast (423) and the right olecranon (430). The vertical side of the first quadrilateral is related to the vertical side of the second quadrilateral by the ratio 1.618:1.0.

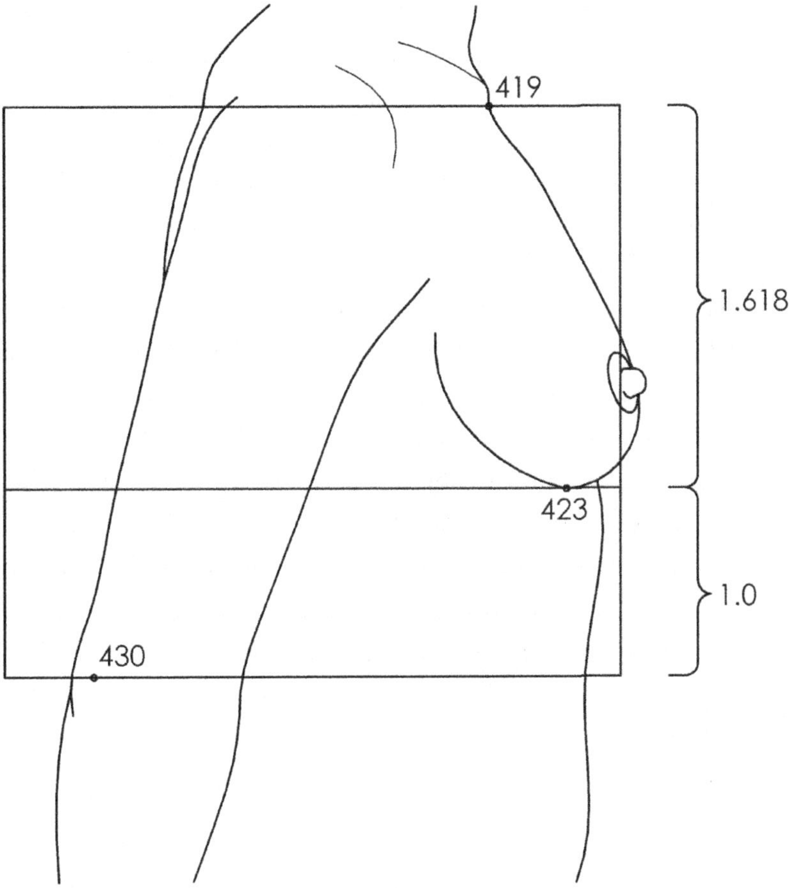

Figure 98. Hayduke Breast Grid 21.

Hayduke Breast Grid 22 (Figure 99) is a grid with three anchor points (anatomic landmarks) that dictate the location of the three horizontal gridlines of this grid. The first anchor point is located at the lowermost inferior border of the left clavicle (424). This point dictates the location of the upper horizontal gridline. The second anchor point is located at the inferior, lowermost, central margin of the left breast (428). This point dictates the location of the middle horizontal gridline. The third anchor point is located at the left olecranon (432). This point dictates the location of the lowermost horizontal gridline. The grid derived from these three anchor points consists of two vertically arranged quadrilaterals. The first quadrilateral is formed between the lowermost inferior border of the left clavicle (424) and the inferior, lowermost, central margin of the left breast (428). The second quadrilateral is formed between the inferior, lowermost, central margin of the left breast (428) and the left olecranon (432). The vertical side of the first quadrilateral is related to the vertical side of the second quadrilateral by the ratio 1.618:1.0.

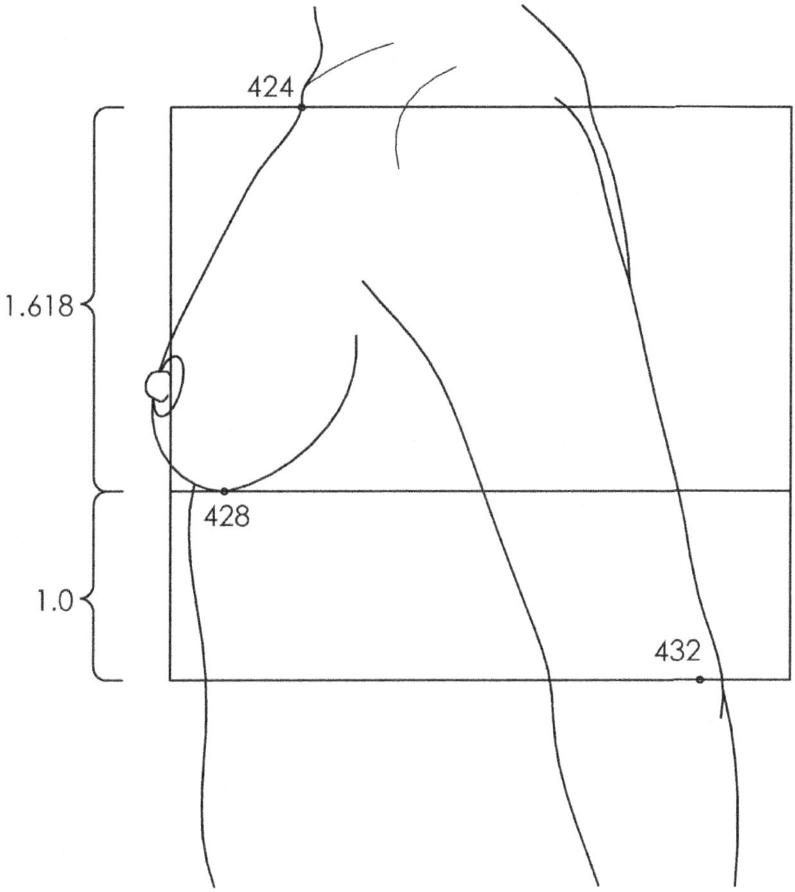

Figure 99. Hayduke Breast Grid 22.

CHAPTER 5

HUMAN BEAUTY ANALYSIS

Past and Current State of the Art

Various methodologies and theoretical components of human physical beauty have been proposed over the years in an attempt to understand human physical attractiveness. Most of the research in this area has been done by evolutionary psychologists who believe that human behavior is largely driven by physical traits that helped our ancestors survive and successfully reproduce. Physical traits that reflect genetic quality or biological fitness are believed to indicate a potential mate's reproductive success.

Mate value is defined as the sum of those traits that are considered desirable in a potential mate. Perceived mate value, in humans, is believed to be partially influenced by the visual appeal of an individual. Evolutionary psychologists believe that certain key components of human facial and body attractiveness underlie assessments of visual appeal and, therefore, mate value. Since some of these key components can be objectively measured, several have been integrated into various attempts at human beauty analysis. Beauty analysis methodologies and theories can be categorized into those that are based upon the neoclassical canons, the averageness hypothesis, symmetry, youthfulness, sexual dimorphism, and the golden ratio.

Neoclassical Canons

Early theories regarding an aesthetically pleasing human appearance were based on the ancient guidelines derived from neoclassical canons of facial and body proportion. The neoclassical canons are descriptions of human proportions that were meticulously recorded by Renaissance period (c. 1300 to 1600) artists. Many of those concepts and guidelines were likely derived from the ancient Greeks (such as Polycleitus) and Romans (such as Vitruvius). One of the most famous neoclassical canon examples is Leonardo da Vinci's drawing that divided the human face into three equal, vertical thirds. These vertical thirds were defined from the bottom of the chin to the bottom of the nose (menton to subnasale), from the bottom of the nose to the eyebrows (subnasale to glabella), and from the eyebrows to the hairline (glabella to trichion) (Figure 100).[1]

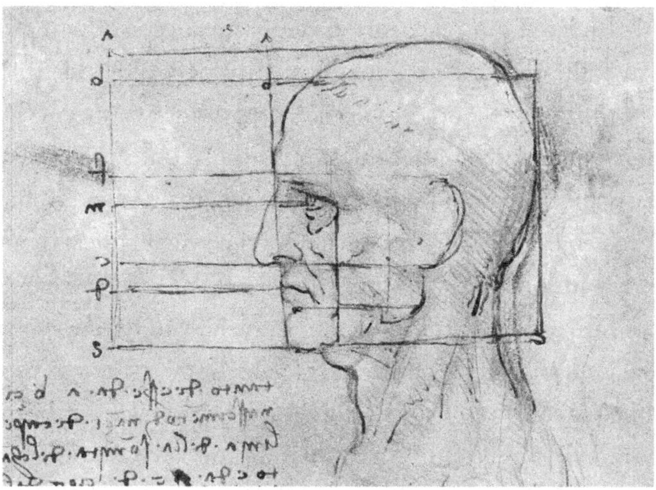

Figure 100. Drawing of the proportions of a head (untitled) by Leonardo da Vinci (c. 1490).

Albrecht Dürer wrote several extended manuscripts on human proportion that were organized and published after his death into a work called *Four Books on Human Proportions* (1528). Dürer dictated, for example, that the distance between the eyes, from the frontal view, should equal the width of one eye.[2] Dürer's entire first two books were detailed descriptions of what he believed to be ideal human proportions (Figures 101 and 102).

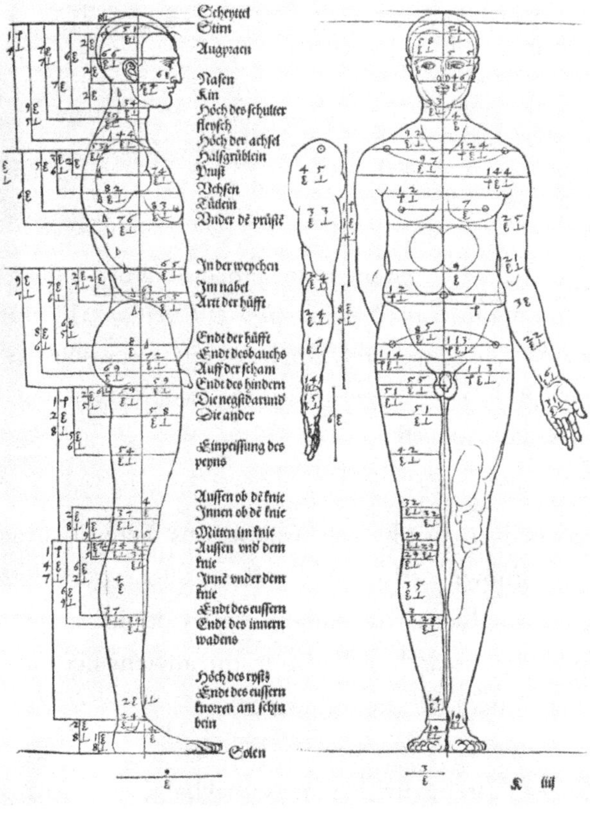

Figure 101. Illustration of the ideal proportions of a male from the *Four Books on Human Proportions* by Durer (1528).

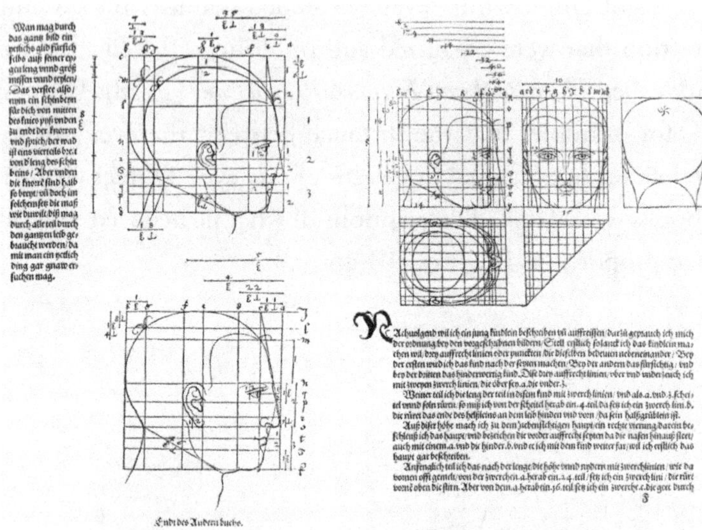

Figure 102. Illustrations of the proportions of a human head from the *Four Books on Human Proportions* by Durer (1528). Durer frequently employed multi-view illustrations of the same body part as a means of representing its three-dimensionality.

Canons of human physical proportions were documented by several lesser known artists of the Renaissance period including Audran, Cousin, Alberti, Savonarla, Pacioli, Cennini, and Francesca.[3] According to the research of Bashour, the ancient neoclassical canons of the face included the following:

1. The head can be divided into equal halves at a horizontal line through the eyes.
2. The face can be divided into equal thirds, with the nose occupying the middle third.

3. The head can be divided into equal quarters, with the middle quarters being the forehead and nose, respectively.
4. The length of the ear is equal to the length of the nose.
5. The distance between the eyes is equal to the width of the nose.
6. The distance between the eyes is equal to the width of each eye (the face width here can be thus divided into equal fifths).
7. The width of the mouth is one and one-half times the width of the nose.
8. The width of the nose is one-fourth the width of the face.
9. The nasal bridge inclination is the same as the ear inclination.
10. The lower face can be divided into equal thirds.
11. The lower face can be divided into equal quarters.[4]

Regarding the modern applicability of ancient neoclassical canons into a meaningful test of beauty and attractiveness, the majority of published research doesn't support their use. The neoclassical canons were originally developed by artists as general guidelines to create a reasonably proportioned human form in their artwork rather than as a true scientific reference of ideal human beauty. Farkas et al. were the first to investigate the validity of nine neoclassical formulas of facial proportions in 153 young adult Caucasians. They also analyzed 308 faces of children at various ages up to age 18. Their analysis didn't support the validity of the neoclassical canons as a universal guide for ideal facial proportions.[3] Other studies tested the applicability of the neoclassical canons to Chinese, Vietnamese, Thai, Turkish, and African-American individuals and arrived at similar conclusions regarding the lack of validity of the neoclassical canons.[5,6,7,8] Although the neoclassical canons may serve well as general guidelines for artists, I do not feel that the neoclassical canons should be applied to modern objective tests of human physical beauty.

Averageness (Arithmetic Mean of Several Faces Morphed Together)

One of the best-known theories regarding human facial beauty is commonly referred to as the "averageness theory" of facial attractiveness. The averageness hypothesis of facial attractiveness has been written about extensively in modern-day psychology literature. Averageness refers to the arithmetic mean of several faces morphed together to create one face that's more beautiful than the original individual component faces. The terms *averageness* and *average* are frequently misleading when used in the context of the averageness hypothesis of facial beauty. Averageness doesn't refer to an "average-looking" face, since the morphed, composite, averaged face is actually more attractive than the individual faces used to create the composite, averaged image.

With modern technology, computer-generated composite faces can be easily created by mathematically averaging (blending, merging, or morphing) multiple individual facial images together to create a single, composite, averaged facial image. This technology has been extensively used in human attractiveness research. For example, researchers mathematically averaged male and female undergraduate students' faces into digitized composite images. Both the composite images and the original images used to make the composites were then judged for attractiveness. The computer-generated, composite, averaged faces were rated by judges as more attractive than the individual component faces used to create the composite images.[9]

The averageness hypothesis contends that averageness seems to be strongly associated with beauty. Rubenstein et al. write in their work describing the role of averageness in defining facial beauty that averageness "is the only characteristic discovered to date that is both necessary and sufficient to ensure facial attractiveness."[10] Langlois, a prominent researcher on the averageness hypothesis, stated, "Based upon our research, we believe that a facial configuration close to the population mean is fundamental to attractiveness."[11] Even research on naturally attractive individuals, such as beauty pageant contestants, has proven that computer-generated averaged composites of the contestants are judged as more attractive than the individual real beauty pageant contestants (Figure 103).[12]

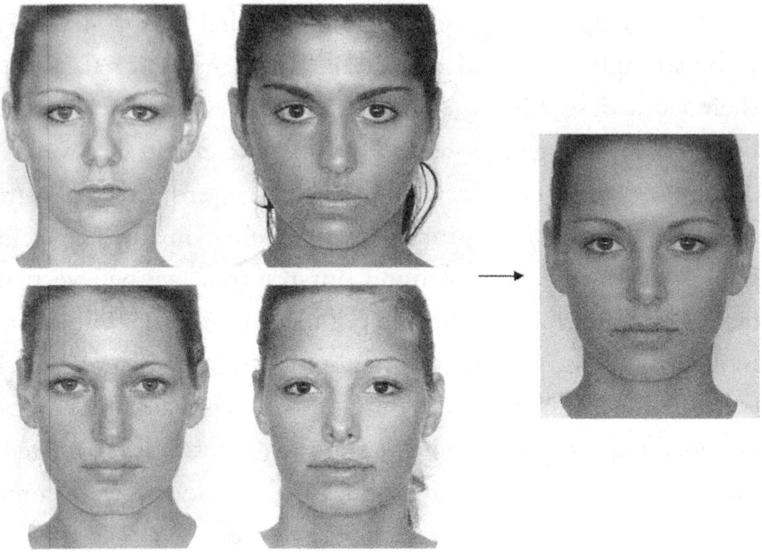

Figure 103. Composite, "averaged" image (far right) computer generated from four Miss Germany beauty pageant contestants (left four images). The computer-generated, composite, "averaged" image was rated as more attractive than any of the faces of the individual women used to create the composite. (Miss Germany beauty pageant contestant images and composite image used with permission of Dr. Martin Gründl.[12])

Rhodes published a large meta-analysis that looked at 20 published studies regarding attractiveness and averageness. Rhodes concluded, "The meta-analysis showed a large effect of averageness on attractiveness (0.52 ± 0.41, M ± SD; 95% CI = 0.42–0.61, N = 45)."[14]

After reviewing the large body of impressive published research on the validity of the averageness hypothesis, I chose to include concepts from the averageness hypothesis in my own beauty analysis methodologies. The design and development stage of many Hayduke Facial Grids involved the use of several, composite, averaged images as references of an ideal facial appearance. As I previously described in Chapter 1, research studies have concluded that, in general, celebrity faces are considered more attractive than noncelebrity faces. In addition, attractive celebrity faces, television actresses, and magazine-cover models were found to have facial proportions and anatomic features that are quite different from human faces that are considered ordinary or unattractive.[1,15]

Within their landmark research publication on the averageness hypothesis, Langlois and Roggman made an intriguing comment regarding the composite, averaged images used in their influential study. They stated, "We also acknowledge that a sample of movie stars might be rated as more attractive than our composites. It may be the case that although averageness is a necessary and critical element of attractiveness, other elements may also be important in influencing judgements of attractiveness."[9] I later applied several concepts from Langlois and Roggman's publication to my grid designs in an attempt to capture those elusive "other elements" that they refer to.

To harness the layout and proportions of the exquisitely attractive facial anatomy of celebrities and movie stars, I merged multiple beautiful faces of celebrities and movie stars into several, composite, averaged images. These composite averaged images were created using software developed by Tiddeman, who developed several innovative computer-graphics methods for psychological and medical facial research.[16,17,18] His software has been used in many published research studies. The composite images that I created with this software were subsequently sharpened by a professional artist and later used as reference images of ideal beauty during the design and development stage of the Hayduke grids. I chose individual component images of celebrities for the composites, which were fully developed young adults not yet affected by the signs of aging. I believe that youthfulness is an important quality to capture when designing reference images of ideal beauty. I specifically targeted the 20- to 28-year-old age range when choosing celebrity photos for the composites to ensure that the qualities of youthfulness existed within my final, morphed composites.

I felt that creating composite, averaged images as reference images of beauty to guide the Hayduke Facial Grid design and development was a superior approach compared to simply using a single facial image of only one model or one actor/actress as a reference image of ideal beauty. I believe that using source images of multiple celebrity faces recognized internationally for their beauty to create averaged, morphed composites was the best option available for creating reference images of ideal facial beauty. Reference images of beauty were absolutely necessary to design the exact anatomic layout of the test grids involved in my beauty analysis methodologies. After much research, I concluded that creating composite, averaged images derived from celebrities who are already considered extremely beautiful in the first place was simply the best approach that modern technology currently offers.

Composite, averaged images of beautiful celebrity faces that were race-specific—such as composite, averaged images of purely Asian faces, purely white faces, and purely black faces—were included in the design and development stage of my test grids. Mixed-race composites of celebrities were also used. When designing reference images of beauty, I felt it was important not to base the design of my test grids on just one race. I believe that factoring in the facial features of beautiful people from multiple races as well as mixed races would yield the highest quality test grids that could be applied to a diverse group of test takers.

Below are just a few examples of the many composite, averaged images that I created as reference images of beauty based on the averageness hypothesis. This is just a small sample of the many composite images used during the Hayduke Grid design and development phase. The examples were created by combining faces of various actresses, celebrities, movie stars, and entertainers known internationally for their stunning beauty. Several of the celebrities used in the morphs were listed in "the most beautiful people in the world" list published by *People* magazine. Some of these celebrities achieved the coveted number-one ranked position on that prestigious list. These celebrities have also been listed on multiple other lists and surveys that consistently recognized them for their physical beauty. Even if someone happens to disagree with a few of the celebrity choices used in my morphed composites, the effect of morphing multiple celebrity images into one composite, averaged image largely negates that issue.

The individual component faces that I used in the white female composite image example that follows included Angelina Jolie, Michelle Pfeiffer, Charlize Theron, Megan Fox, Keira Knightley, and Amber Heard (Figure 104). The individual component faces used in the black female composite image example included Vanessa Williams, Rhianna (Fenty), Tyra Banks, Beyoncé (Knowles-Carter), Zoe Saldana, and Kerry Marisa Washington (Figure 105). The individual component faces used in the Asian female composite image example included Nana (Im Jin-ah), Irene (Bae Joo-hyun), Fan Bingbing, Wang Feifei, Zhang Zilin, and Lee Young-ae (Figure 106). The mixed-race female composite image was derived from all of the above eighteen individuals combined (Figure 107).

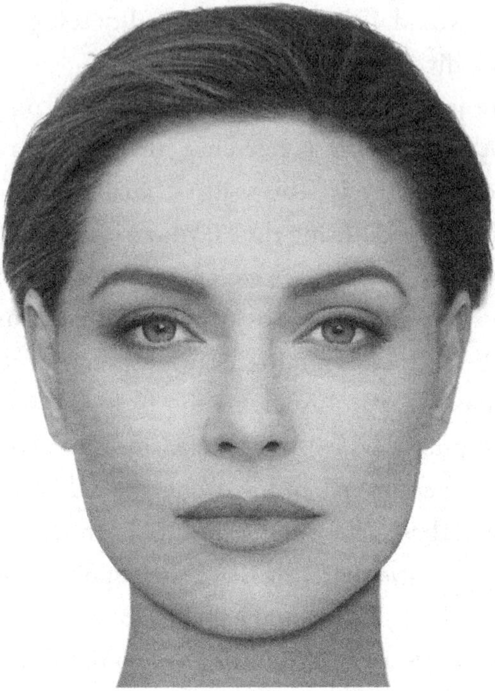

Figure 104. White, female, composite, averaged image derived from the faces of Angelina Jolie, Michelle Pfeiffer, Charlize Theron, Megan Fox, Keira Knightley, and Amber Heard. This is one of the composite, averaged, reference images of beauty used during the design and development stage of the Hayduke Facial Grids.

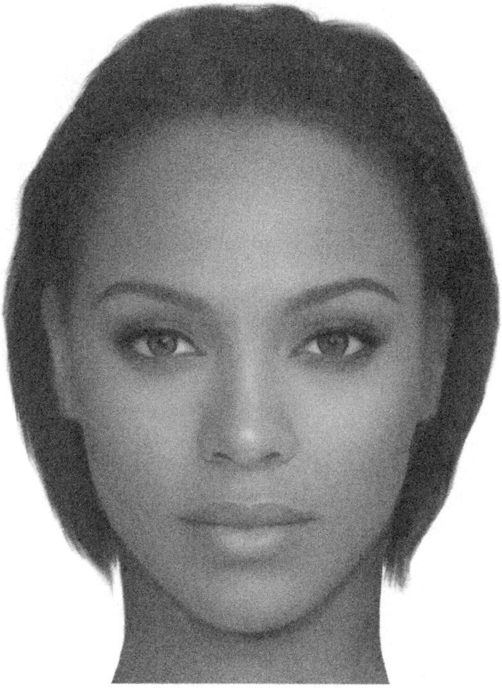

Figure 105. Black, female, composite, averaged image derived from the faces of Vanessa Williams, Rhianna (Fenty), Tyra Banks, Beyoncé (Knowles-Carter), Zoe Saldana, and Kerry Marisa Washington. This is one of the composite, averaged reference images of beauty used during the design and development stage of the Hayduke Facial Grids.

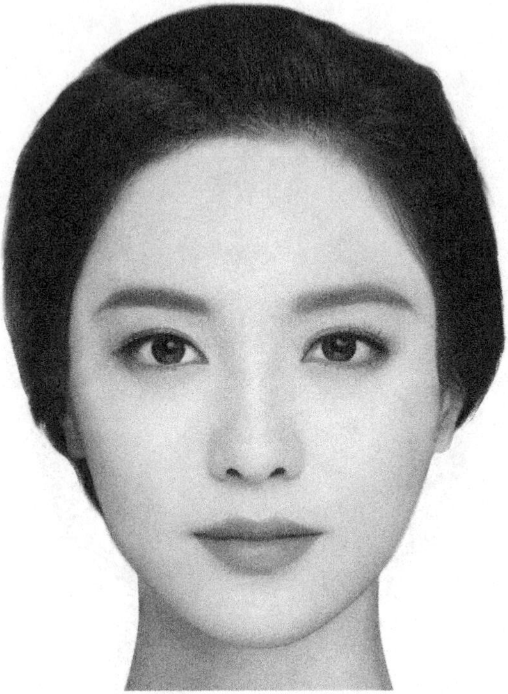

Figure 106. Asian, female, composite, averaged image derived from the faces of Nana (Im Jin-ah), Irene (Bae Joo-hyun), Fan Bingbing, Wang Feifei, Zhang Zilin, and Lee Young-ae. This is one of the composite, averaged reference images of beauty used during the design and development stage of the Hayduke Facial Grids.

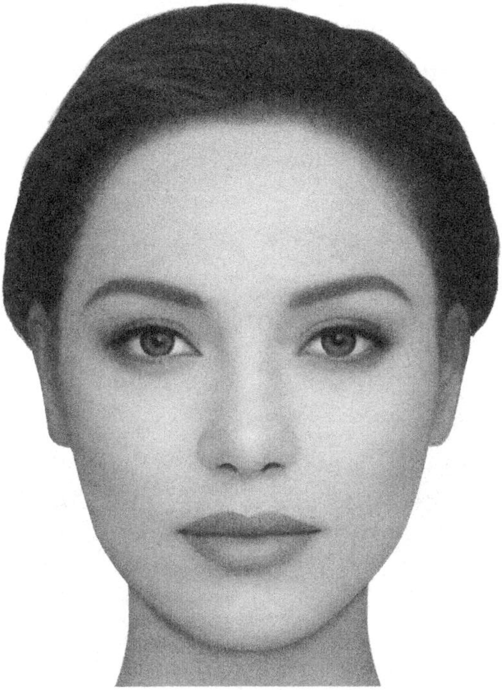

Figure 107. Mixed-race, female, composite, averaged image derived from mixing the faces used in the white female, black female, and Asian female composite images. Eighteen faces from three races were used to create this particular mixed-race composite image. This is one of the composite, averaged reference images of beauty used during the design and development stage of the Hayduke Facial Grids.

Composite, averaged images of males from multiple races as well as mixed races were also created and used in the design and development phase of my grids. The identical approach of using individual component celebrity faces of males who are well recognized for their physical attractiveness was used to create the male composites. Figure 108 depicts an example of a white, male composite image derived from the faces of David Beckham, Johnny Depp, Brad Pitt, Chris Hemsworth, Chris Pine, and Sean O'Pry.

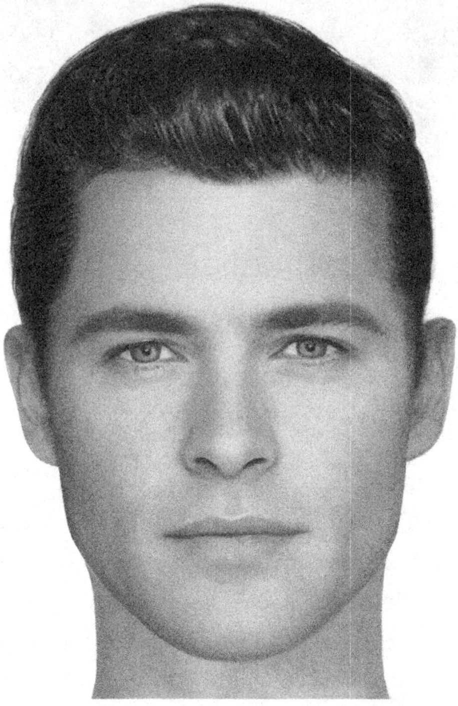

Figure 108. White, male, composite, averaged image derived from the faces of David Beckham, Johnny Depp, Brad Pitt, Chris Hemsworth, Chris Pine, and Sean O'Pry. This is one of the male, composite, averaged reference images used during the design and development phase of the Hayduke Facial Grids.

Symmetry

Some analytical methods of facial beauty are based on the symmetry hypothesis. The symmetry hypothesis contends that symmetrical faces are more attractive than asymmetrical faces. Symmetrical faces are those where the right and left sides of the face look identical. Asymmetrical faces have anatomic differences between the right and left sides of the face. Perrett's study concluded that "increasing symmetry of face shape increases ratings of attractiveness for both male and female faces."[19] Grammer and Thornhill also concluded in their study that human facial attractiveness ratings were influenced in a positive way by facial symmetry.[13]

Rhodes researched the association of facial symmetry with attractiveness in non-Western cultures. She created computer-generated, perfectly symmetrical versions of Japanese faces and compared them to the true natural versions of the exact same faces—which were naturally somewhat asymmetrical. Raters preferred the computer-generated, perfectly symmetrical versions over the real-life asymmetrical versions of the same Japanese face. Rhodes concluded that the preference for symmetry in faces also applies to non-Western cultures and that this preference for symmetry in the human face is biologically based.[20]

Rhodes also studied symmetry in Caucasian faces. She created four versions of the same face with varying levels of symmetry. Symmetry levels were categorized as low, normal, high, and perfectly symmetrical. She found that ratings of attractiveness increased as symmetry increased and decreased when symmetry was decreased[21] (Figures 109 and 110).

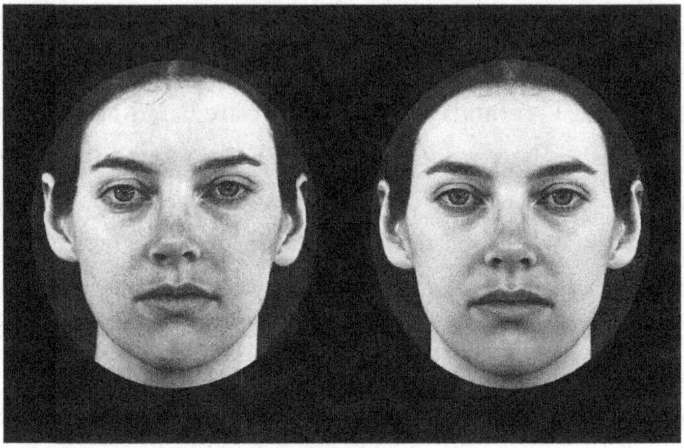

Figure 109. Example of a low-symmetry image (left) next to a perfectly symmetrical image (right) of the same face used in Rhodes' research. The image on the left has definite differences between the levels of her eyes and between the two sides of her face. Raters preferred the perfectly symmetrical version (right). (Image used with permission of Dr. Gillian Rhodes)

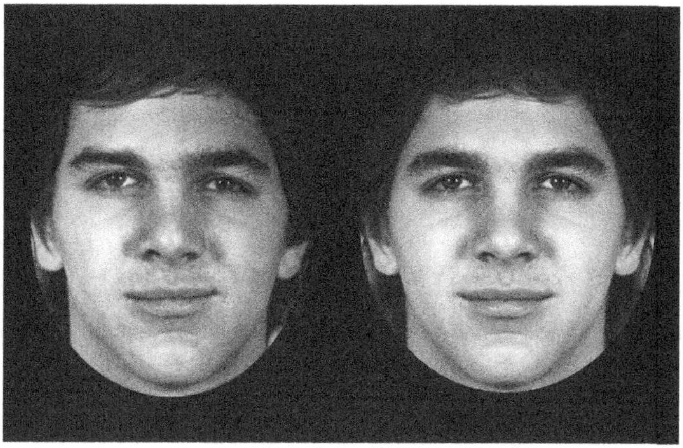

Figure 110. Example of a low-symmetry image (left) next to a perfectly symmetrical image (right) of a male face used in Rhodes' research. Notice the difference between the levels of his eyes, nostrils, and mouth in the low-symmetry image (left) compared to the perfectly symmetrical image (right). Raters preferred the perfectly symmetrical image on the right. (Image used with permission of Dr. Gillian Rhodes)

Another interesting study by Kowner found that raters preferred symmetrical faces in images of elderly people much more so than in the faces of young people. Kowner believed that this preference for symmetry in elderly faces "may be because symmetry serves as a cue for youth in old age".[22] He believed that the soft-tissue changes of the face that occur with aging possibly lead to increasing asymmetries in the human face with time. Sutton found that asymmetry of certain human facial features, such as the nose, seem to worsen significantly with age.[23]

As a plastic surgeon, I find it obvious that symmetry between right- and left-sided anatomic features is very important to attractiveness, but absolute perfect symmetry is not. Concepts of symmetry apply to human anatomic structures that have both right- and left-sided elements, such as eyes, nostrils, eyebrows, ears, lips, jaws, cheekbones, and breasts. I believe that small degrees of asymmetry (differences) between the right and left sides of the face or breasts is aesthetically acceptable and actually quite normal. Minor asymmetries don't seem to have a negative impact on the perceived beauty of an individual. Many people who are recognized internationally for their outstanding facial beauty frequently have slight asymmetries between the right and left sides of their face. These subtle facial asymmetries aren't noticed by the general public, since they're usually quite minor.

Choi asked 434 medical students to evaluate photos of women's faces and found that small asymmetries within the face weren't noticed by the judges. Choi concluded that "images with canting and differences less than 3°–4° and 3–4 mm, respectively, are generally not recognized as asymmetry."[24] Clearly, some anatomic asymmetry is indeed acceptable and generally goes unnoticed. For this reason, my testing methods within the Hayduke Facial Analysis test and Hayduke Breast Analysis test allow for a certain degree of acceptable asymmetry. The degree of acceptable asymmetry allowed in my facial and breast tests can be custom set within the Divine Face® and Divine Breasts® software settings.

Youthfulness

Youthfulness, in general, is considered an integral component in attractive human faces and breasts. Including elements of youthfulness in beauty analysis methodologies is intuitive and clearly appropriate. Research has established that, after a certain age, getting older is generally associated with progressively decreasing attractiveness. The only adult age range where there doesn't seem to be a meaningful relationship between increasing age and decreasing attractiveness is between the ages of 18 and 30 years.[10,25] During this narrow time period, humans are fully physically mature but not yet old enough to show negative signs of aging. For this reason, I feel that this particular age range (18 to 30 years old) is the proper age range to target when creating reference images of ideal beauty for beauty analysis methodologies.

Many published studies have described decreasing facial attractiveness as being associated with increasing age.[26,27,28,29,30] Maestripieri et al. researched the ratings of facial attractiveness in two specific age groups of women and men that he considered middle-aged (35 to 50 years old and 51 to 65 years old). As many others have concluded, he found a negative association with aging and facial attractiveness. In addition, however, his results also showed that the decrease in facial attractiveness rating for the 51-to-65-year-old group for women (postmenopausal group) was significantly worse than for the 35-to-50-year-old age group.[31] I found his study particularly interesting, since age 50 seems to be the most common age at which many of my patients, especially females, seek out my services for facial age-reversing surgical procedures. Although facial aging changes are usually not dramatic at age 50, facial aging changes seem to become noticeable and bothersome to many females around that particular age.

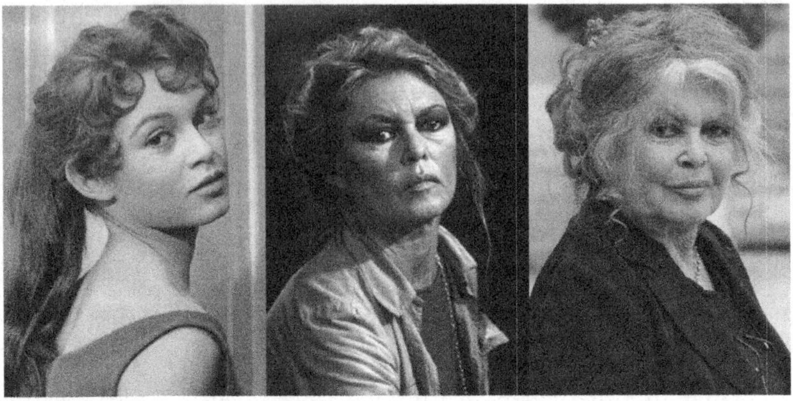

Figure 111. Images of French actress Brigitte Bardot at various ages, exemplifying the natural aging process of the face and neck. Age 20 (left), age 53 (middle), and age 72 (right). In the most youthful image (left), her neck skin is tight, her jawline borders are very well-defined and her eyebrows are in a high, attractive location.

Palm Springs, California, is primarily a retirement community (median age of 54) where the pursuit of a refreshed, youthful appearance via plastic surgery is quite common. Because of the demographics, cosmetic plastic surgery—facelifts, necklifts, eyelid rejuvenation, and browlifts—to reverse the signs of aging is a frequent request by my "over-50" Palm Springs clientele. Loose, sagging skin under the chin, excess upper eyelid skin, and jowling at the jawline are among the most frequent facial aging complaints that I hear. Injectable agents are also very popular in this age group. Female lips, due to the pubertal effects of estrogen, surprisingly reach their fullest appearance between 14 and 15 years of age.[32] Aging female lips appear thinner (older), and the pursuit of youthfulness has sparked the popularity of injectable agents that plump up the lips to a fuller appearance. Unfortunately, overzealous injection of fillers into the lips and cheeks is quite common and creates an unbalanced, "over-stuffed" facial appearance that can be quite unsightly. Conservative injection of filler material, however, to create a subtle improvement in lip definition can be very attractive, even in younger females in their mid 30s and 40s. The quest to regain wrinkle-free, smooth, youthful facial skin via laser skin resurfacing, chemical peels or botulinum toxin injections is also common in my over-50 clientele.

Some researchers believe that youthfulness in an adult face is associated with facial characteristics that are commonly seen in early childhood—such as small noses and large eyes (as related to the rest of the face). Cunningham published a study on female facial beauty that examined the results of 50 adult female photographs rated by men. He found that small noses, large eyes, and high eyebrows in an adult female's face were positively associated with physical attractiveness.[33] My personal practice of plastic surgery definitely supports these findings. Patients in my plastic surgery practice who are unhappy with their noses most commonly voice a request for a smaller nose. My Beverly Hills office clientele, who tend to be either in the entertainment industry or aspire to be in the entertainment industry, frequently seek out smaller noses. To this day, I've never heard any of my Beverly Hills patients voice a request for a bigger nose.

Higher eyebrows in females are pursued either with endoscopic (minimally invasive) browlift surgery or non-surgically by simply having eyebrows professionally shaped or tattooed to give the impression of a slightly higher, youthful eyebrow location. Non-surgical tricks that are frequently used to give the impression of larger (wider) eyes include curling the eyelashes, brushing eyebrows upwards, applying lengthening mascara, and hiding dark circles (shadows) under the eyes with light-colored concealer makeup. All of these pursuits, both surgical and non-surgical, attempt to address a desire for the youthful female facial characteristics of large eyes and high eyebrows.

Regaining a youthful breast appearance is also one of the most frequent requests in any plastic surgeon's practice, including my own. Aging breasts are generally characterized by drooping of the nipples to a low position on the breast mound, lengthening of the entire breast (sometimes beyond the umbilicus), flattening of the upper half of the breast, and widening of the areolas. Patients who are unhappy with the aged appearance of their breasts pursue plastic surgery to achieve a higher position of their nipples, narrower areolas, shortening of the breasts' length (to counteract a droopy appearance), and a fuller (less flat) upper-breast contour. The goal of breast surgery in patients with aging breasts is to regain the characteristics of a youthful breast—or at least an improvement toward youthful breast characteristics.

Sexual Dimorphism (the Degree of Femininity and Masculinity of Anatomic Features)

Some believe that the degree of femininity and masculinity of human facial features is linked to the degree of facial attractiveness in a human face. Setting aside the obvious differences in the sexual organs themselves, the differences in other characteristics between the two sexes of the same species define the term *sexual dimorphism*.

Testosterone is thought to affect human male faces in puberty by causing several distinct physical changes. The degree of these masculine changes varies widely among males and determines how masculine the male's face will appear in adulthood. Under the effects of testosterone, those particular pubertal boys who are genetically destined to develop masculine facial features will experience widening of the jawbone (mandible) and cheekbone area. The brow ridge (bony prominence of the forehead just above the eye sockets) enlarges and protrudes forward. The chin enlarges, and the entire lower face lengthens. The jaw may develop a square, "manly" appearance. The eyebrows thicken and the lips thin. The eyes develop a somewhat sunken, "deep-set" appearance and become relatively narrow (small) compared with the rest of the face. The eyebrows descend to a lower position on the forehead as compared with an average or non-masculine male face. Hollywood tends to cast actors with the most extreme masculine facial features in stereotypical "tough guy" roles (Figure 111). Actors with these types of extremely masculine facial features include Ron Perlman (*Hellboy, Sons of Anarchy*), Danny Trejo (*Machete*), Jason Momoa (*Game of Thrones*), Dwayne "The Rock" Johnson (*Hercules*), Jason Statham (*Killer Elite, The Mechanic*), Charles Bronson (*Death Wish*), Sylvester Stallone (*Rocky, Rambo*) and Richard Kiel (who played "Jaws" in several *James Bond* franchise films).

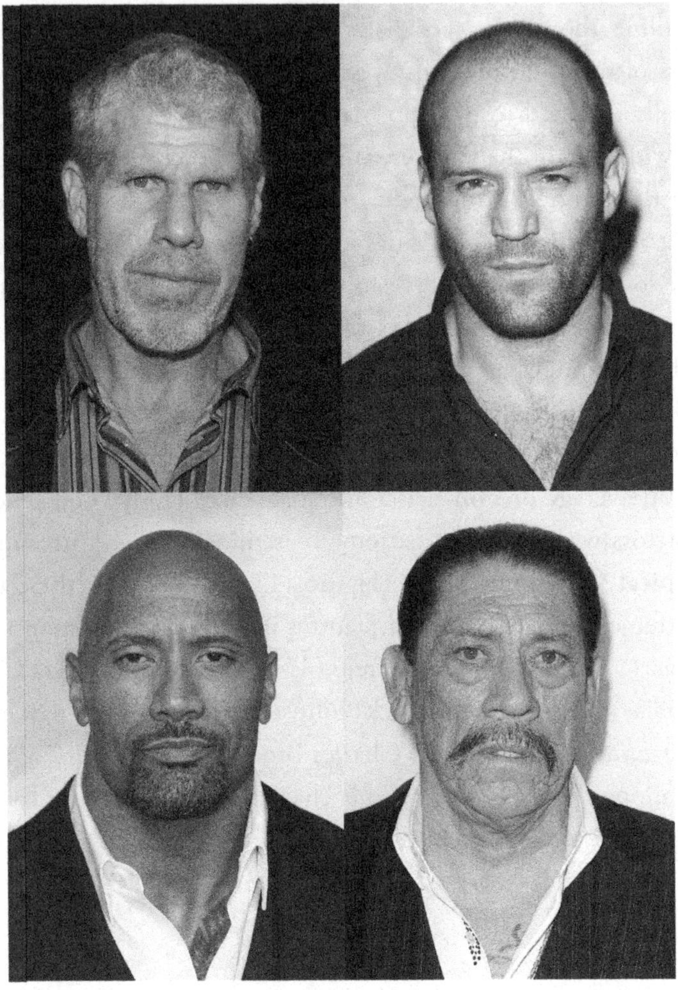

Figure 112. Actors with extremely masculine facial features who are frequently cast in "tough guy" roles. Ron Perlman (upper left), Jason Statham (upper right), Dwayne "The Rock" Johnson (lower left), and Danny Trejo (lower right). Masculine features include large jaws, tall chins, protruding forehead brow ridges and low eyebrows.

Estrogen is the key hormone involved in the development of feminine features in females during puberty. The degree of femininity in a female's face varies widely among women. Female faces that possess a high degree of femininity will generally display quite high and prominent cheekbones. The eyebrows will be positioned high on the forehead, and the eyebrows themselves will be thin. The facial skin will be hairless and smooth. The length of a feminine jaw will be short and somewhat narrow in width compared to males. The eyes will appear wide (large) and the lips will appear full (thick). Estrogen also increases fat deposition into the female breast and hip regions. This results in larger (more feminine) breasts and hips.

Research supports the concept that femininity in the female face is highly correlated with attractiveness.[13] Several studies have even found that when feminine features are exaggerated, they actually further increase rated attractiveness.[34,35,36,37,38] The effects of masculine traits on a male's facial attractiveness aren't as clear. Some studies have shown a positive correlation of ratings of masculinity with attractiveness in men, but this correlation wasn't as strong as femininity with attractiveness in women.[39,40,41,42] In fact, some research has shown a preference for feminized male faces rather than masculine male faces.[36,37,43] It's been suggested that the relationship between masculinity and attractiveness may be curvilinear in males, with moderate masculinity being more desirable than extreme masculinity.[39] Certainly, enough controversy exists in the published literature regarding masculinity and attractiveness that caution should be exercised when including components of extreme masculinity in any objective test of male facial beauty. I believe that incorporating elements of moderate masculinity in male facial analysis methodologies is the most prudent approach.

Golden Ratio Relationships within Human Anatomic Features

Compared to all of the other methodologies and theories regarding beauty analysis described in this chapter, I contend that testing for golden ratio relationships between individual features of an anatomic area is the optimal method upon which to base an objective aesthetic evaluation of the human face and breasts. The golden ratio is perhaps the most ubiquitous, controversial, and mysterious proportion related to beauty, harmony, and attractiveness in the history of mankind. Countless books and articles have described the golden ratio as it relates to the beautiful appearance of many physical objects. Although it's not the only element involved in human physical beauty, I believe that the golden ratio's presence in the layout of human facial and breast features provides the true foundation for the eye-appealing appearance present in those fortunate individuals who we perceive as physically beautiful. I believe that the greater the number of golden ratio relationships that exist within an individual's anatomic features, the more likely it is for that particular individual (or for that particular anatomic area) to be perceived as physically beautiful.

As I've previously described, the discovery of the golden ratio itself is commonly attributed to the brilliant ancient mathematicians Pythagorus of Samos (c. 570–c. 495 BC) and Euclid of Alexandria (c. 325–c. 265 BC). It is believed that many sculptors, painters, and artists since that time have attempted to apply the golden ratio to achieve beautiful, harmonious, human anatomic proportions in their artwork. As far as a true clinical application of the golden ratio by health care professionals to treat patients, there have been surprisingly few published descriptions in the literature.

Despite knowledge of the ratio's existence since ancient times, use of the golden ratio in health care has been minimal.

Two clinical applications of the golden ratio by health care professionals have been described in the fields of dentistry and oral maxillofacial surgery. Levin, a dentist, applied the golden ratio to the aesthetics of human teeth by creating a golden ratio–based dental grid.[44] This grid, printed on a small, disposable piece of paper, can be inserted into the patient's mouth at the time of dental treatment. The appearance of the eight front upper teeth are believed to be the most important for both an attractive smile and a natural dental appearance. Levin's dental grid dictates that, in properly proportioned front upper teeth, the width of the largest front upper tooth (central incisor) is related to the width of the immediately adjacent smaller tooth (lateral incisor) by the golden ratio. This golden ratio relationship continues with the width of the lateral incisor and the adjacent smaller tooth (canine). The width of the canine is related to the immediately adjacent tooth (first premolar) with the same golden ratio relationship. Levin also believes that the total width of the lips in an attractive smile (from lip corner to lip corner) should be in golden proportion to the combined width of the front eight upper teeth. Levin's dental grid has found clinical utility in guiding the aesthetics of dental crowning procedures of the frontal teeth in which a cap is permanently glued over a damaged tooth to restore the tooth's size, shape, and strength.

Marquardt, an oral maxillofacial surgeon, invented a golden decagon overlay mask in an attempt to assess human facial features within a single, large mask that encompassed the entire face. Marquardt contends that his mask, created in the 1990s, is a representation of an idealized form of the human face. This mask is based on a complex golden decagon matrix structure, which was derived from the golden ratio. Marquardt's mask has clinical utility as a guide for orthodontic treatment.[45] Bashour scientifically evaluated Marquardt's mask and concluded that Marquardt's mask, "is a first step in producing an objective system for measuring facial attractiveness."[46]

Holland later published research in a peer-reviewed journal that criticized Marquardt's mask. Holland wrote, "The mask also appears to approximate the face shape of masculinized European women."[47] Holland maintained that Marquardt's mask doesn't fit sub-Saharan African and East Asian faces, nor does it reflect an attractive, feminized, female face of any race. Focusing on the premise that it's been well established by a large body of published research that above average femininity in a female's face is considered more attractive by the general public,[13] Holland felt that fitting Marquardt's masculine-appearing mask shouldn't be a goal for white women seeking cosmetic surgery. Holland went on to say that "Marquardt's mask does not appear to describe an 'ideal' face shape, even for white women, because its proportions are inconsistent with the optimal preferences of most people, especially with regard to femininity."[47]

Implementation of Golden Ratio Test Grids in Surgical Planning

Compared to prior published attempts at a clinical analysis of human anatomy that incorporated the golden ratio, I strived to achieve a method that is both easier to visually understand and to apply. My method also allows for a more precise targeting of specific, independent, anatomic areas within the face and breasts. I strived for a user-friendly and minimalistic design within both the

Hayduke Facial Analysis and Hayduke Breast Analysis tests. The approach I used to create multiple reference images of ideal human anatomic features included composite, averaged images of attractive people recognized internationally for their beauty. My tests are applicable to test takers from multiple races as well as mixed races. I selectively included several fundamental concepts and elements in my tests from the large body of previously published, peer-reviewed literature regarding the essential key components of human physical beauty and attractiveness. I believe that using multiple, strategically placed small grids within a single test yields a more precise anatomic analysis compared with trying to create one large overlay grid or one large mask that encompasses the entire anatomic area (such as the entire face) all at once.

Although my testing methods are primarily based on golden ratio relationships within human anatomic features, the golden ratio isn't the sole element involved in my methodologies. I believe that a truly meaningful test of beauty requires inclusion of several key components and concepts derived from peer-reviewed scientific publications on human physical beauty. *Symmetry* is a significant component within many of the grids involved in my tests—specifically, within those grids that simultaneously include both the right and left sides of the chest or face within the same grid. In addition, *composite, averaged images* were used to create several reference images of ideal beauty involved in the design and development phase of many of my test grids. These composite, averaged images used as beauty references also included race-specific composites of people recognized internationally for their facial beauty within their own racial group. This included composite, averaged images of purely Asian faces, purely black faces, and purely white faces. Mixed-race reference composites were also utilized in my reference grid creation process. Separate male and female composite, averaged images were also created as gender-specific beauty references. The universally recognized traits of *youthfulness* were also an integral part of the reference images used in the design phase of both my facial and breast grids. My facial and breast analysis methodologies involve a blend of all of these various elements of human physical beauty, with the golden ratio functioning as the core underlying component.

Although the core Hayduke Facial Grids were designed to apply to a diverse range of races and ethnicities, several customized Hayduke Facial Grids and test modifications were created to account for the consistent anatomic differences that exist between beautiful people of different races, ethnicities, and genders. Examples of these consistent anatomic differences include the shorter lower facial height (shorter jaw) that's considered beautiful in an Asian female's face as compared to the relatively longer lower facial height (slightly taller jaw) that's considered beautiful in a white female's face. The attractive Asian face is also wider as measured from the outer edges of the cheekbones (zygomas) compared with the narrower facial width characteristic of attractive white and black faces. Race-specific grids that account for the wider nasal width, nostrils, and lips of the beautiful black face were also created. Custom grids and test modifications to address issues of this nature are essential to achieve an ethnically and racially appropriate evaluation of human anatomic facial features. Several grids and test modifications that account for anatomic gender differences between male and female faces were also created. Attractive male faces, for example, consistently possess lower and flatter (less-arched) eyebrows, thinner lips, and larger (taller) jaws as compared with attractive female faces. In order for customized grids and appropriate test modifications to be applied during the Hayduke Facial Analysis test, users are given the option to input race, ethnicity, and gender within the Divine Face® application software.

Precise targeting of individual, small areas of the face or breasts—rather than the entire face or entire breast area—is another unique feature of my tests. The ability to do so is relevant for surgeons who are specifically working on only one small area within the face or breasts. Since the Hayduke Facial Analysis and Hayduke Breast Analysis tests are both composed of a battery of individual grids that evaluate zones (segments) within the face and breasts, relevant grids can be tested over the specific areas of interest. For example, if browlift surgery or blepharoplasty (eyelid cosmetic surgery) is planned, the surgeon may choose to test the patient with facial grids that only include the eyelids and eyebrows. If lip injections are planned for lip rejuvenation, grids that only include lips can be tested.

After the test grids are applied, the "failed" grids that didn't comply with a golden ratio anatomic layout are closely analyzed. In some cases, a failed grid can serve as an excellent guide for the physician's treatment plan. In the case of cosmetic plastic surgery, the ultimate goal for the physician would be to convert a failed grid into a "successful" grid with some type of intervention that changes the patient's anatomy (e.g., surgery, cosmetic filler injection, etc.).

The section that follows illustrates several examples of the clinical application of Hayduke Facial Grids and Hayduke Breast Grids in my own personal practice of plastic surgery. The Hayduke Facial Grids and Hayduke Breast Grids used in these examples were converted from failed grids to successful grids after I performed plastic surgery on the test takers (i.e., patients).

The patient in Figures 113 and 114 presented to me with complaints about her peri-ocular appearance. She complained of low, "intense"-appearing eyebrows that were making her eyes and face look older than her true age. The anatomic landmarks that define Hayduke Facial Grid 15 include landmarks at the eyebrow arch peak, upper eyelid margin, and lower eyelid margin. Pre-operative (before surgery) testing of this patient's face with Hayduke Facial Grid 15 achieved a failed result because of the low position of her eyebrows in relation to her upper and lower eyelid margins. The pre-operative ratio created within the defined landmarks of Hayduke Facial Grid 15 for this patient was 1.15:1.0, which was scored as a failed grid on the Hayduke Facial Analysis test. This grid also has a symmetry component, since this grid requires that anatomic landmarks of both the right and left sides of the face be horizontally level (within a certain reasonable percentage, set as the allowable "tilt offset" value within the Divine Face® application software).

After browlift surgery, this patient's eyebrows and forehead were raised upwards. This anatomic change slightly enlarged the vertical side of the upper quadrilateral component of Hayduke Facial Grid 15. The new measurements after surgery, between the same anatomic landmarks, achieved a ratio within Hayduke Facial Grid 15 of 1.618:1.0 (Figure 113). This grid was now scored as a successful grid. On the Hayduke Facial Analysis test, this patient just improved her overall score because of targeted, plastic surgical intervention on a small, isolated facial area.

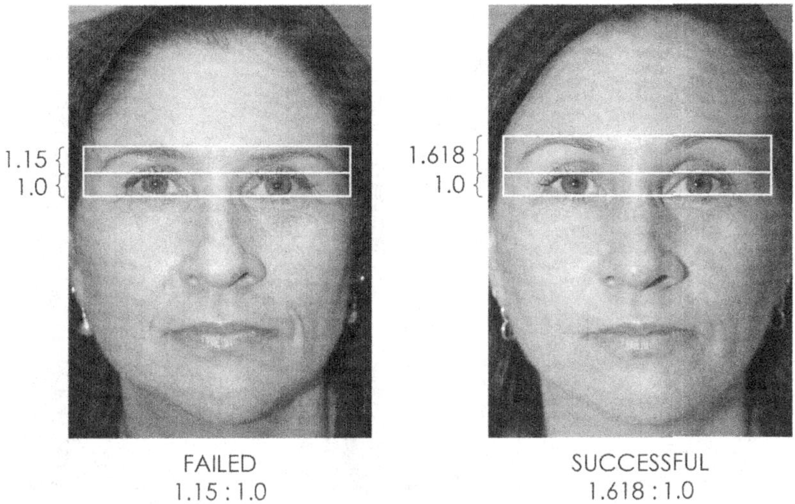

Figure 113. Hayduke Facial Grid 15 applied before (left) and after (right) browlift surgery. After Dr. Andrew J. Hayduke performed browlift surgery, this patient's eyebrows were elevated to a more youthful position. Plastic surgery converted a "failed" grid into a "successful" grid. The 1.618:1.0 ratio was achieved in this grid after plastic surgery because the relationships between the anatomic landmarks of this grid were improved by browlift surgery. (Actual patient of Andrew J. Hayduke, M.D.)

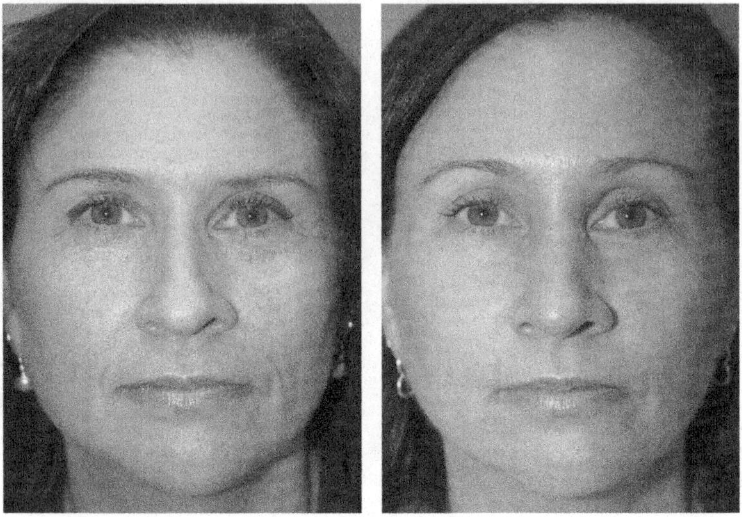

Figure 114. Before (left) and after (right) images following a surgical browlift performed by Andrew J. Hayduke, M.D. Hayduke Facial Grid 15 was used during pre-surgical planning. (Actual patient of Andrew J. Hayduke, M.D.)

The gentleman in Figures 115 and 116 presented to me with complaints about the appearance of his nose. He felt that the tip of his nose was "too big" and ball-like. Pre-operative testing of his nose with Hayduke Facial Grid 22 revealed a failed result. The ratio created between the anatomic landmarks of Hayduke Facial Grid 22 resulted in a ratio of 0.93:1.0 (fail). I sculpted the cartilage of his nasal tip during cosmetic rhinoplasty to create a smaller and more refined nasal tip. After surgery, retesting with Hayduke Facial Grid 22 revealed a ratio of 1.618:1.0 between the identical anatomic landmarks of this grid. The grid was now scored as successful on re-testing after cosmetic surgery. Rhinoplasty created a smaller, more refined nasal tip that achieved a golden ratio relationship between the anatomic landmarks of Hayduke Facial Grid 22. After surgery, his nose seemed to blend more harmoniously with the rest of his facial features.

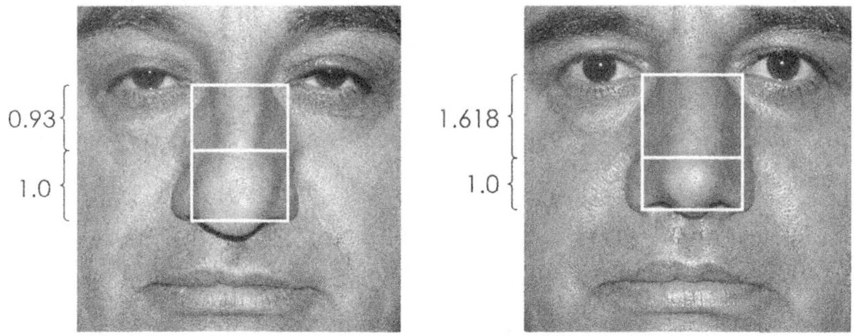

Figure 115. Hayduke Facial Grid 22 applied before (left) and after (right) cosmetic rhinoplasty. Before surgery, this patient failed Hayduke Facial Grid 22, since the ratio within the grid was 0.93:1.0. After cosmetic rhinoplasty, retesting of the same patient with Hayduke Facial Grid 22 revealed a new ratio of 1.618:1.0 since his anatomy was changed by cosmetic surgery. (Actual patient of Andrew J. Hayduke, M.D.)

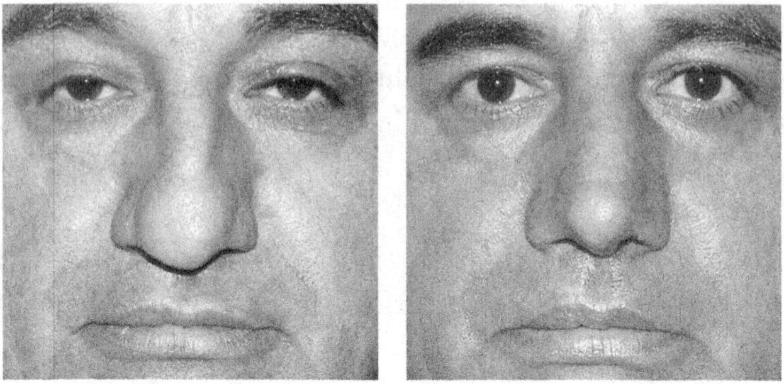

Figure 116. Appearance before (left) and after (right) cosmetic rhinoplasty by Andrew J. Hayduke, M.D. After surgery, this gentleman's nose blends more harmoniously with the rest of his facial features. Testing with Hayduke Facial Grid 22 was used to plan his cosmetic rhinoplasty. (Actual patient of Andrew J. Hayduke, M.D.)

The patient in Figures 117, 118, and 119 presented to me with complaints of a droopy, deflated breast appearance with wide areolas. She complained that her breasts looked much older than her actual age, and she was very self-conscious about their appearance. She had several prior breast surgeries performed by other plastic surgeons and was still very dissatisfied with her breasts. Multiple Hayduke Breast Grids were used to plan her complex cosmetic breast surgery. Before surgery, the ratio between the anatomic landmarks of Hayduke Breast Grid 14 from left profile view revealed a ratio of 3.2:1.0 (fail). I elevated her nipple areolas to a higher position and improved the droopy appearance of her breasts with a cosmetic mastopexy (breast lift). I also decreased the overall size (diameter) of her areolas. I improved the fullness and shape of her deflated-appearing upper breast area with conservatively sized breast implants.

She wanted to maintain a small, conservative breast size. Retesting with Hayduke Breast Grid 14 after cosmetic surgery resulted in a ratio of 1.618:1.0 between the same anatomic landmarks (Figure 117). After cosmetic surgery, her breasts (from multiple views) blend harmoniously with the rest of her body and have a youthful, more attractive appearance (Figures 117,118, and 119).

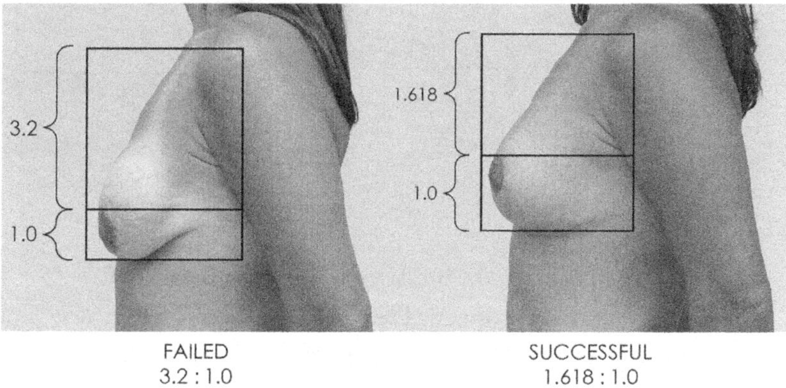

Figure 117. Hayduke Breast Grid 14 applied before (left) and after (right) cosmetic mastopexy combined with breast augmentation. Before surgery (left), this patient failed Hayduke Breast Grid 14, since the ratio within the grid was 3.2:1.0. After surgery (right), the anatomy of the breast was changed, and a successful fit of Hayduke Breast Grid 14 was achieved. (Actual patient of Andrew J. Hayduke, M.D.)

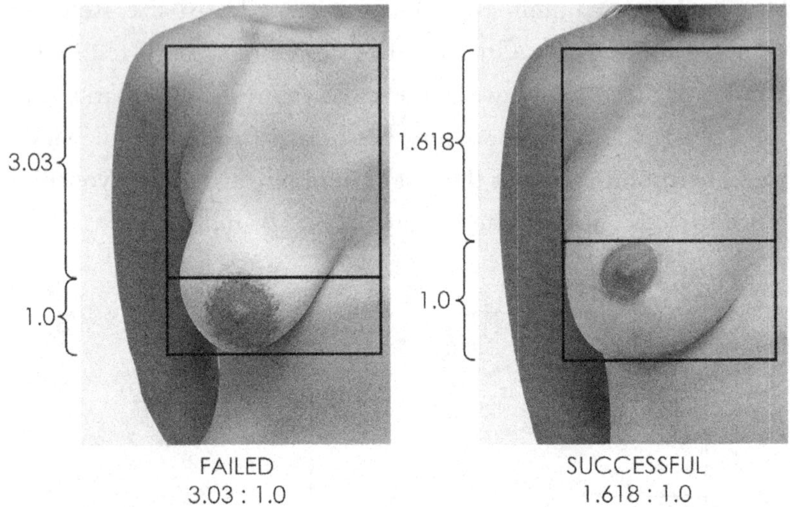

Figure 118. Hayduke Breast Grid 5 applied before (left) and after (right) cosmetic breast surgery. Testing with Hayduke Breast Grid 5 revealed a "failed" result before surgery with a ratio of 3.03:1.0. After surgery, a ratio of 1.618:1.0 was achieved between the anatomic landmarks that define Hayduke Breast Grid 5. After the anatomic changes of cosmetic surgery, Hayduke Breast Grid 5 was scored as "successful." (Actual patient of Andrew J. Hayduke, M.D.)

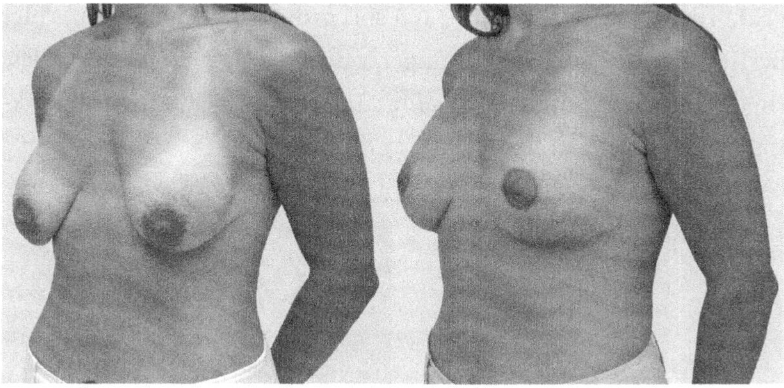

Figure 119. Appearance of the same patient as in Figures 117 and 118 before (left) and after (right) cosmetic breast surgery. Her surgical plan was devised with the assistance of several Hayduke Breast Grids. After surgery, her breasts and nipple areolas appear youthful and significantly more attractive. She wanted to maintain small, conservatively sized breasts. (Actual patient of Andrew J. Hayduke, M.D.)

The patient in Figures 120 and 121 presented to me with complaints of low eyebrows, forehead wrinkling, and an overall undesirable, aged appearance of her eyes. She also wanted the aging changes of her jawline and neck tastefully improved upon without the stigmata of overdone facial plastic surgery. Before surgery, testing her peri-ocular area with Hayduke Facial Grid 36 resulted in a ratio of 1.157:1.0, which was scored as a failed grid by the Hayduke Facial Analysis test. Based on that result, I formulated a surgical plan to raise her eyebrows and forehead slightly upwards. After endoscopic browlift surgery, retesting with Hayduke Facial Grid 36 revealed a new ratio of 1.618:1.0 between the landmarks of this grid. This grid was now score as a successful grid (Figure 120). Her peri-ocular area appeared younger, refreshed, less intense, and less tired after plastic surgery. Facelift surgery achieved a natural-looking improvement in her jawline and neck.

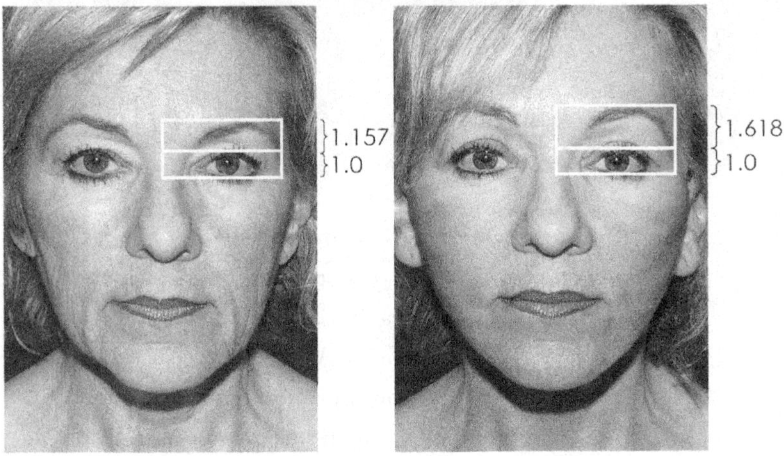

FAILED
1.157 : 1.0

SUCCESSFUL
1.618 : 1.0

Figure 120. Hayduke Facial Grid 36 tested both before (left) and after (right) browlift and facelift surgery by Andrew J. Hayduke, M.D. Before surgery, this patient failed Hayduke Facial Grid 36. After browlift surgery, a "successful" fit of this grid was achieved. (Actual patient of Andrew J. Hayduke, M.D.)

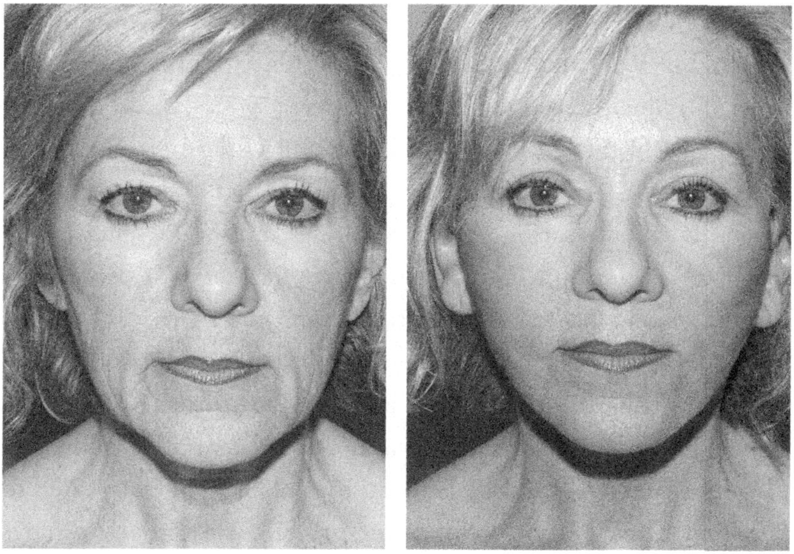

Figure 121. Facial appearance before (left) and after (right) undergoing an endoscopic browlift, blepharoplasty, and facelift by Andrew J. Hayduke, M.D. Hayduke Facial Grid 36 was used during her pre-surgical planning. The facelift achieved a more refined jawline as well as an effective elevation of her cheeks (midface). Cheek implants were not used. This patient appears youthful, less intense, and refreshed after surgery, without an artificial, "plastic" appearance. The amount of eyebrow elevation was carefully planned with the help of several Hayduke Facial Grids used as pre-surgical guides. (Actual patient of Andrew J. Hayduke, M.D.)

The patient in Figures 122 and 123 presented to me with significant differences in the appearance of her two breasts (breast asymmetry). Her right nipple areola was in a dramatically lower position compared with her left nipple areola, best seen in Figure

123. Her entire right breast drooped lower compared with her left breast. The right and left areolas were of different diameters (Figure 123). She also requested a larger overall breast size, especially an increase in the fullness of the upper half of her breasts. She felt that the upper half of her breasts appeared flat and unfeminine, especially when wearing bathing suits and certain low-cut dresses. Pre-operative testing with multiple Hayduke Breast Grids was performed to help devise her cosmetic surgical plan. The surgical plan was to perform a right-sided breast lift (mastopexy) to address the droopy asymmetric right breast and to insert breast implants on both sides to address the size, shape, and volume of both breasts. Hayduke Breast Grids that included the golden spiral were used to help guide her final breast implant size. Figure 122 demonstrates the utility of Hayduke Breast Grid 16 in revealing the deficit in size and shape of the left breast before surgery (white arrows). Analyzing the amount of breast-size deficit before surgery helped guide the choice of breast implant size that would ultimately agree with the attractive golden ratio anatomic relationships of Hayduke Breast Grid 16. Her pre-operative appearance and final surgical results are also shown in Figure 123.

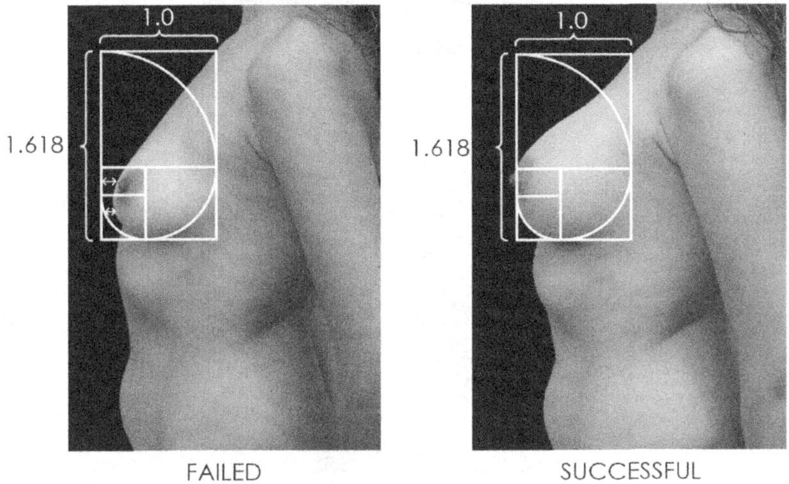

Figure 122. Hayduke Breast Grid 16 applied before (left) and after (right) cosmetic breast augmentation (breast implant surgery). This grid consists of a golden rectangle with a golden spiral within the golden rectangle. Before surgery (left), the front of this patient's breast did not extend to the front of the golden rectangle (white arrows) and the bottom of the breast did not follow the shape of the golden spiral within Hayduke Breast Grid 16. After surgery (right), the increased size and improved shape derived from the breast implant surgery (breast augmentation) allowed the breast to extend to the front of the golden rectangle and to follow the gentle, lowermost curve of the golden spiral within Hayduke Breast Grid 16. After surgery (right), this grid was scored as a "successful" fit on Hayduke Breast Analysis testing. (Actual patient of Andrew J. Hayduke, M.D.)

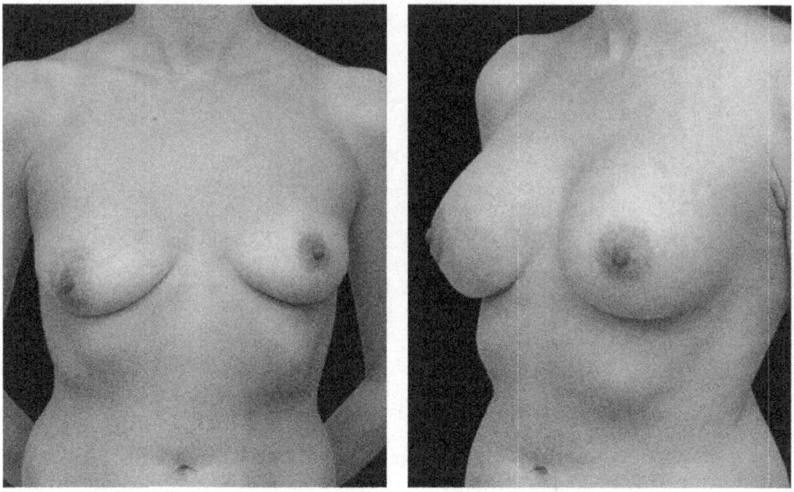

Figure 123. Breast appearance before (left) and after (right) cosmetic breast surgery. This patient had significant differences (asymmetries) between her two breasts. Multiple Hayduke Breast Grids were used before surgery to help plan her complex cosmetic breast surgery. Hayduke Breast Grids that included the golden spiral were used to help choose her final breast implant size. This patient underwent a right-sided mastopexy (breast lift) and breast implant insertion (breast augmentation) on both sides. Before (left) and after (right) images are shown. After surgery (right), her nipple areolas are at the same level and both breasts have a fuller, more attractive, feminine appearance that blends harmoniously with her chest, shoulders, and abdomen. (Actual patient of Andrew J. Hayduke, M.D.)

The patient in Figures 124 and 125 presented to me with complaints of a small (retrusive) chin. She didn't like her facial appearance from the profile view. Before surgery, testing with Hayduke

Facial Grid 35 revealed a failed result with a grid ratio of 0.38:1.0 (Figure 124). I formulated a surgical plan to enlarge her chin with a chin implant (facial implant). After chin implant surgery, retesting with Hayduke Facial Grid 35 revealed a ratio of 1.618:1.0. The grid was now scored as a successful grid. After surgery, her profile appears more balanced, and her new, larger chin blends harmoniously with rest of her facial features (Figure 125).

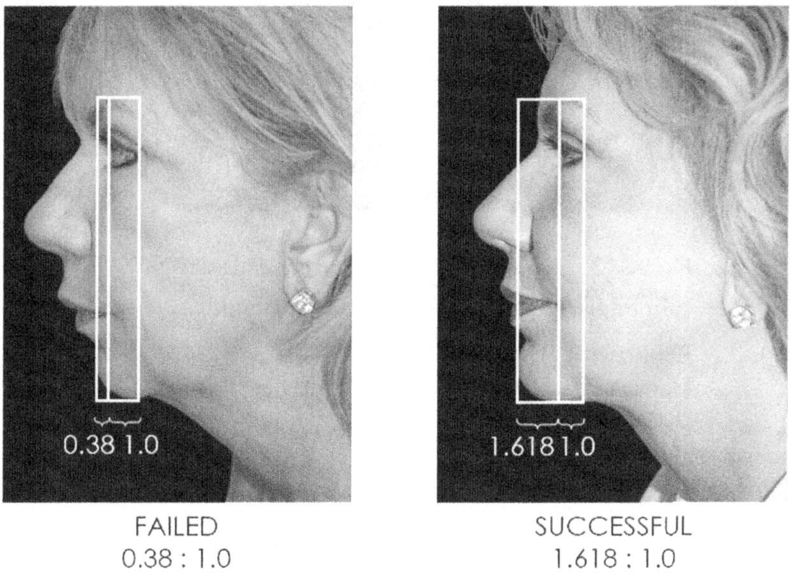

Figure 124. Hayduke Facial Grid 35 tested both before (left) and after (right) chin implant surgery by Andrew J. Hayduke, M.D. Before surgery, this patient failed Hayduke Facial Grid 35. Chin implant surgery enlarged the chin and achieved a 1.618:1.0 ratio within this grid. (Actual patient of Andrew J. Hayduke, M.D.)

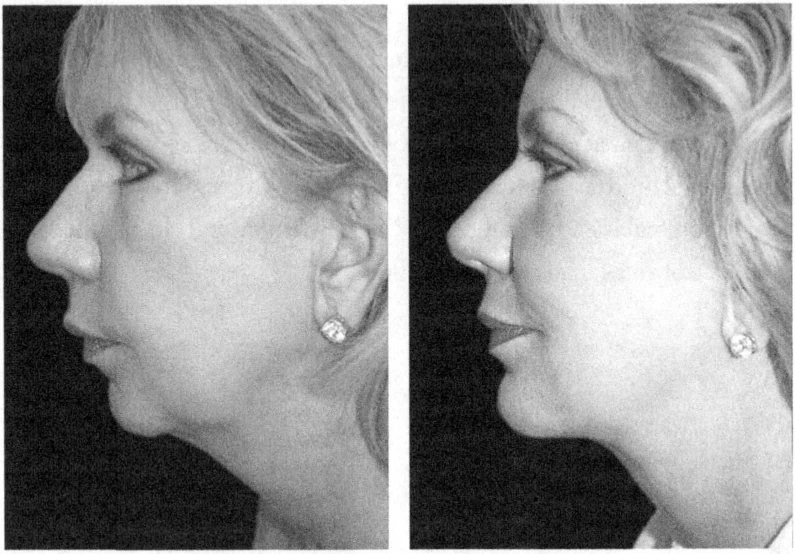

Figure 125. Appearance before (left) and after (right) chin implant surgery. The facial balance and harmony improved significantly after chin implant surgery. Hayduke Facial Grid 35 helped formulate this patient's pre-surgical plan. (Actual patient of Andrew J. Hayduke, M.D.)

As I've just demonstrated, my approach to anatomic feature analysis can potentially serve as a guide for plastic surgical planning before surgery or to evaluate surgical results after surgery. My methods can also be used to objectively evaluate beauty pageant contestants, professional fashion models, and actors/actresses for the presence of the visually appealing anatomic qualities found in golden ratio relationships. These tests may also help to objectively predict success in pursuits that are highly dependent upon an attractive physical appearance, a task that was previously delegated to guessing. In addition, lay people who aren't involved in any of these endeavors may simply find it interesting to see how well their face or breasts would score in an objective beauty analysis test.

Attempting to test for beauty within human anatomic features is an extremely difficult undertaking. Beauty analysis methodologies will always be met with opposition and criticism from the scientific community. As I've described in detail in Chapter 1 of this treatise, a substantial amount of research has disproved the commonly heard adage, "Beauty is in the eye of the beholder." Unfortunately, most people outside academic psychology circles have simply not read the relevant research regarding the objective nature of human physical beauty. Despite all the published scientific evidence demonstrating that human physical beauty is indeed an objective and universal quality, it seems that controversy regarding this concept will always exist.

Rapidly evolving advances in computer technology, improved software algorithms, and highly detailed photographic image capture technologies have allowed me to create what I hope is considered a reasonable approach to an objective testing of human facial and breast beauty. I've drawn pertinent concepts from the large body of previously published research on human physical beauty as well as from modern computer science technologies to create the Hayduke Facial Analysis and Hayduke Breast Analysis tests.

I believe that *golden ratio* relationships between human anatomic features function as the underlying foundation of a beautiful human physical appearance. I also believe that golden ratio relationships work synergistically with several other essential key components of human physical beauty. These complementary, essential components include *youthfulness,* a certain degree of anatomic *symmetry,* and physical features that resemble the arithmetically *aver-*

aged appearance of composite images derived from people who are universally accepted as physically beautiful. By combining all of these elements within the Hayduke Facial Analysis and Hayduke Breast Analysis tests, I believe that my methodologies offer a meaningful assessment of the aesthetics of the human face and breasts.

REFERENCES

CHAPTER 1: OBJECTIVITY AND SCIENCE WITHIN BEAUTY — MERGING OF PHILOSOPHY, ART, AND MATHEMATICS

[1] Beauty. Merriam-Webster Dictionary. https://www.merriam-webster.com. Accessed October 1, 2019.

[2] Aesthetics. Merriam-Webster Dictionary. https://www.merriam-webster.com. Accessed October 1, 2019.

[3] Berlyne DE. *Studies in the New Experimental Aesthetics.* New York, NY: John Wiley & Sons; 1974.

[4] Lewicki P. *Nonconscious Social Information Processing.* New York, NY: Academic Press; 1986.

[5] Veryzer RW Jr. Aesthetic response and the influence of design principles on product preferences. In: McAliser L, Rothschild ML, eds. *NA – Advances in Consumer Research.* Vol. 20. Provo, UT: Association for Consumer Research; 1993:224–228.

[6] Badr L, Abdallah B. Physical attractiveness of premature infants affects outcome at discharge from the NICU. *Infant Behavior and Development.* 2001;24:129–133. doi: 10.1016/S0163-6383(01)00068-6

[7] Langlois JH et al. Maxims or myths of beauty? A meta-analytic and theoretical review. *Psychological Bulletin.* 2000;126(3):390–423.

[8] Buss DM. *Evolutionary Psychology: The New Science of the Mind.* Boston, MA: Allyn & Bacon; 1999.

[9] Daly M. Evolutionary theory and parental motives. In: Krasnegor NA, Bridges RA, eds. *Mammalian Parenting.* New York: Oxford University Press; 1990.

[10] Mann J. Nurturance or negligence: maternal psychology and behavioral preference among preterm twins. In: Barkow JH, Cosmides L, Tobby J, eds. *The Adapt Mind: Evolutionary Psychology and the Generation of Culture*. New York, NY: Oxford University Press; 1992:367–390.

[11] Barden RC et al. Effects of craniofacial deformity in infancy on the quality of mother-infant interactions. *Child Development.* 1989;24:819–824.

[12] Daly M, Wilson M. Discriminative parental solicitude and the relevance of evolutionary models to the analysis of motivational systems. In: Gassaniga MS, ed. *The Cognitive Neurosciences.* Cambridge, MA: MIT Press; 1995:1269–1286.

[13] Stephan CW, Langlois JH. Baby beautiful: adult attributions of infant competence as a function of infant attractiveness. *Child Development.* 1984;55:576–585.

[14] Epps S. Labeling effects of infant health and parent demographics on nurses' ratings of preterm infant behavior. *IMHJ* (University of Nebraska Medical Center). 1993:14(3):182–191.

[15] Vaughn BE, Langlois JH. Physical attractiveness as a correlate of peer status and social competence in preschool children. *Developmental Psychology.* 1983;19:561–567.

[16] Langlois JH, Stephan C. The effects of physical attractiveness and ethnicity on children's behavioral attributions and peer preferences. *Child Development.* 1977;48:1694–1698.

[17] Stephan CW, Langlois JH. Physical attractiveness and ethnicity: implications for stereotyping and social development. *Journal of Genetic Psychology.* 1980;137:303–304.

[18] Dion KK. Physical attractiveness and evaluations of children's transgressions. *Journal of Personality and Social Psychology.* 1972;24(2): 207–213.

[19] Dion KK, Berscheid E, Walster E. What is beautiful is good? *Journal of Personality and Social Psychology*. 1972;24(3):285–290.

[20] Ambady N, Rosenthal R. Half a minute: predicting teacher evaluations from thin slices of nonverbal behavior and physical attractive-

ness. *Journal of Personality and Social Psychology.* 1993;64:431–441.

[21] Adams GR, Cohen AS. Children's physical and interpersonal characteristics that affect student-teacher interactions. *The Journal of Experimental Education.* 1974;43:1–5.

[22] Clifford MM, Walster E. Research note: the effect of physical attractiveness on teacher expectations. *Sociology of Education.* 1973;46:238–258.

[23] Rich J. Effects of children's physical attractiveness on teacher's evaluations. *Journal of Educational Psychology.* 1975;67:599–609.

[24] Langlois JH, Styczynski LE. The effects of physical attractiveness on the behavioral attributions and peer preferences of acquainted children. *International Journal of Behavioral Development.* 1979;2:325–341.

[25] Krantz M. Physical attractiveness and popularity: a predictive study. *Psychological Reports.* 1987;60:723–726.

[26] Watkins L, Johnston L. Screening job applications: the impact of physical attractiveness and application quality. *International Journal of Selection and Assessment.* 2000;8:76–84.

[27] Cash TF, Gillen B, Burns SD. Sexism and beautyism in personnel consultant decision making. *Journal of Applied Psychology.* 1977;62(3):301–310.

[28] Marlowe CM, Schneider SL, Nelson CE. Gender and attractiveness biases in hiring decisions: are more experienced managers less biased? *Journal of Applied Psychology.* 1986;81(1):11–21.

[29] Harper B. Beauty, stature, and the labour market: a British cohort study. *Oxford Bulletin of Economics and Statistics.* 2000;62:771–800.

[30] Saporta I, Halpern JJ. Being different can hurt: effects of deviation from physical norms on lawyers' salaries. *Industrial Relations.* 2002;41(3):442–466.

[31] Maccarone D. Affirmative action for the attractive. *Psychology Today.* 2003;36(1):8.

[32] Hamermesh D, Biddle J. Beauty and the labor market. *American Economic Review.* 1994;84:1174–1194.

[33] Darby BW, Jeffers D. The effects of defendant and juror attractiveness on simulated courtroom trial decisions. *Social Behavior and Personality: An International Journal.* 1988;16(1):39–50.

[34] Downs AC, Lyons PM. Natural observations of the links between attractiveness and initial legal judgments. *Personality and Social Psychology Bulletin.* 1991;17:541–547.

[35] McKelvie SJ, Coley J. Effects of crime seriousness and offender facial attractiveness on recommended treatment. *Social Behavior and Personality: An International Journal.* 1993;21(4):265–277.

[36] Vrij A, Firmin HR. Beautiful thus innocent? The impact of defendants' and victims' physical attractiveness and participants' rape beliefs on impression formation in alleged rape cases. *International Review of Victimology.* 2001;8(3):245–255.

[37] Mazzella R, Feingold A. The effects of physical attractiveness, race, socioeconomic status, and gender of defendants and victims on judgments of mock jurors: a meta-analysis. *Journal of Applied Social Psychology.* 1994;24:1315–1344.

[38] Walster E et al. Importance of physical attractiveness in dating behavior. *Journal of Personality and Social Psychology.* 1966;4:508–516.

[39] Townsend JM, Levy GD. Effects of potential partners' physical attractiveness and socioeconomic status on sexuality and partner selection. *Archives of Sexual Behavior.* 1990;19:149–164.

[40] Highest-Paid Models 2018: Kendall Jenner Leads With $22.5 Million. Forbes. https://www.forbes.com/sites/natalierobehmed/2018/12/13/highest-paid-models-2018-kendall-jenner-leads-with-22-5-million/#228c22b3ddf1. Published December 12, 2018. Accessed November 1, 2019.

[41] Plato, *Philebus*, 51B.

[42] Aristotle, *Poetics*, volume 2, 2322. [1450b34]

[43] Aristotle, *Metaphysics*, volume 2, 1705. [1078a36]

[44] Stobaeus, *Eclogues.* IV 1.40 H, frg. D4, Diels.

[45] Plato, *Sophist*, 228 A.

[46] Pollio MV. *On Symmetry: In Temples and in the Human Body*, Book 3, Chapter 1.

[47] Alberti LB. De Statua. In: Janitschek H, ed. *Leone Battista Albertis kleinere kunsttheoretische Schriften*. Vienna, Austria: W. Braumüller; 1877.

[48] Hume D. *Of the Standard of Taste*. 1757

[49] Ginsborg H. Kant's aesthetics and teleology. In: Zalta EN, ed. *The Stanford Encyclopedia of Philosophy*. 2014. https://plato.stanford.edu/archives/fall2014/entries/kant-aesthetics/.

[50] Di Dio C, Macaluso E, Rizzolatti G. The golden beauty: brain response to classical and renaissance sculptures. *PLoS ONE*. 2007;2(11): e1201. doi: 10.1371/journal.pone.0001201

[51] Shen H. Brain responses to facial attractiveness induced by facial proportions: evidence from an fMRI study. *Scientific Reports*. 2016;6:35905. doi: 10.1038/srep35905

[52] Nedeljkovic N. Evaluation of facial beauty using anthropometric proportions. *Scientific World Journal*. 2014; article ID 428250. http://dx.doi.org/10.1155/2014/428250

[53] Ferrario V. Facial morphometry of television actresses compares with normal women. *J Oral Maxillofac Surg*. 1995;53:1008–1014.

[54] Rupesh S, Rakesh J, Winnier J, et al. The role of the divine proportion in the perception of beauty: a cross sectional study. *Amrita Journal of Medicine*. Jan–Jun 2014;10(1):1–44.

[55] Pancherz H, Knapp V, Erbe C, Heiss AM. Divine proportions in attractive and nonattractive faces. *World J Orth*od. Spring 2010;11(1):27–36.

[56] Coetzee V, Greeff J, Stephen I, Perrett D. Cross-cultural agreement in facial attractiveness preferences: the role of ethnicity and gender. *PLoS One*. 2014;9(7):e99629. https://doi.org/10.1371/journal.pone.0099629

[57] Cunningham MR, Roberts AR, Barbee AP, Druen PB, Wu C-H. Their ideas of beauty are, on the whole, the same as ours: consistency and variability in the cross-cultural perception of female physical attractiveness. *Journal of Personality and Social Psychology.* 1995;68(2):261–279. http://dx.doi.org/10.1037/0022-3514.68.2.261

[58] Zebrowitz LA, Wang R, Bronstad PM, Eisenberg D, Undurraga E, Reyes-García V, Godoy R. (2012). First Impressions from faces among U.S. and culturally isolated Tsimane people in the Bolivian rainforest. *Journal of Cross-Cultural Psychology.* 2012;43(1):119–134. https://doi.org/10.1177/0022022111411386

[59] Langlois J, Kalakanis L, Rubenstein A, Larson A, Hallam M, Smoot M. Maxims or myths of beauty? A meta-analytic and theoretical review. *Psychological Bulletin.* 2000;126(3):390–423. doi: 10.1037/0033-2909.126.3.390

CHAPTER 2: ALL THAT GLITTERS IS GOLD — FUNDAMENTALS OF THE GOLDEN RATIO

[1] Stampler L. How much the world's most iconic logos cost companies to design. *Business Insider.* March 25, 2013. https://www.businessinsider.com/heres-how-much-the-worlds-most-iconic-logos-cost-companies-2013-3.

[2] Kleiner F. *Gardner's Art Through the Ages: A Global History.* 15th ed. Boston, MA: Cengage Learning; 2016.

[3] Connelly J. *The Parthenon Enigma: A New Understanding of the West's Most Iconic Building and the People Who Made It.* New York, NY: Vintage Books; 2014.

[4] Doczi G. *The Power of Limits: Proportional Harmonies in Nature, Art, and Architecture.* Boulder, CO: Shambhala Publications; 1981.

[5] Lund F. *Ad Quadratum: A study of the Geometrical Bases of Classic and Medieval Religious Architecture, with Special Reference to Their Application in the Restoration of the Cathedral of Nidaros (Throndhjem), Norway.* Pranava Books; 2019.

[6] Clark L, director. *Donald in Mathmagic Land.* Los Angeles: Walt Disney Productions; 1959.

[7] Le Corbusier. *The Modulor*, 2nd ed. Cambridge, MA: Harvard University Press; 1958.

[8] Activity: Golden Ratio. Museum of Science, Boston, MA (website). https://www.mos.org/leonardo/activities/golden-ratio

[9] McGucken E. *The Golden Number Ratio Principle: Why the Fibonacci Numbers Exalt Beauty and How to Create Phi Compositions in Art, Photography, and Design.* 45EPIC Golden Hero's Odyssey Mythology; 2016.

[10] Densmore D, ed. *Euclid's Elements.* Santa Fe: Green Lion Press; 2002.

[11] Cook T. *The Curves of Life.* Mineola, NY: Dover Publications; 1979.

[12] Tsuji K, Muller S. *Spirals and Vortices in Culture, Nature, and Science.* New York: Springer Publishing; 2019.

CHAPTER 3: DIVINE FACE — BEAUTY ANALYSIS OF THE HUMAN FACE BASED ON THE GOLDEN RATIO

[1] Hayduke AJ. System and method for analyzing features of a human face using one or more overlay facial grids. US patent 9,721,146. August 1, 2017.

[2] Hayduke AJ. System and method for analyzing features of a human face using one or more overlay facial grids. US patent 9,996,943. June 12, 2018.

[3] DiBernardo BE, Adams RL, Krause J, Fiorillo MA, Gheradini G. Photographic standards in plastic surgery. *Plast Reconstr Surg.* 1998;102:559–568.

CHAPTER 4: DIVINE BREASTS — BEAUTY ANALYSIS OF THE HUMAN BREAST BASED ON THE GOLDEN RATIO

[1] Hayduke AJ. U.S. Patent Application No. 16593126. 2019.

[2] DiBernardo BE, Adams RL, Krause J, Fiorillo MA, Gheradini G. Photographic standards in plastic surgery. *Plast Reconstr Surg.* 1998;102:559–568.

CHAPTER 5: HUMAN BEAUTY ANALYSIS — PAST AND PRESENT STATE OF THE ART

[1] Milutinovic J, Zelic K, Nedeljkovic N. Evaluation of facial beauty using anthropometric proportions. *Scientific World Journal.* 2014;2:428250.

[2] Farkas LG, Kolar JC. Anthropometrics and art in the aesthetics of women's faces. *Clin Plast Surg.* 1987;14:599.

[3] Farkas LG, Hreczko TA, Kolar JC, et al. Vertical and horizontal proportions of the face in young adult North American Caucasians: revision of neoclassical canons. *Plast Reconstr Surg.* 1985;75:328–338.

[4] Bashour M. History and current concepts in the analysis of facial attractiveness. *Plast Reconstr Surg.* October 2006;118(3):741–756.

[5] Le TT, Farkas LG, Ngim RC, Levin LS, Forrest CR. Proportionality in Asian and North American Caucasian faces using neoclassical facial canons as criteria. *Aesthetic Plast Surg.* 2002: 26:64–69.

[6] Wang D, Qian G, Zhang M, Farkas LG. Differences in horizontal, neoclassical facial canons in Chinese (Han) and North American Caucasian populations. *Aesthetic Plast Surg.* 1997;21:265–269.

[7] Jayaratne YS, Deutsch CK, McGrath CP, Zwahlen RA. Are neoclassical canons valid for southern Chinese faces? [published ahead of print December 28, 2012]. *PLoS One.* 2012;7(12):e52593. doi: 10.1371/journal.pone.0052593

[8] Borman H, Ozgur F, Gursu G. Evaluation of soft-tissue morphology of the face in 1,050 young adults. *Ann Plast Surg.* 1999;42:280–288.

[9] Langlois JH, Roggman LA. Attractive faces are only average. *Psychol Sci.* 1990;1(2):115–121.

[10] Rubenstein AJ, Langlois JH, Roggman LA. What makes a face attractive and why: the role of averageness in defining facial beauty. In: Rhodes G, Zebrowitz L, eds. *Facial Attractiveness, Advances in Visual Cognition.* Vol. 1. Norwood, NJ: Ablex; 2002:1–33.

[11] https://labs.la.utexas.edu/langloislab/face-perception/the-beauty-of-averageness/. Accessed July 29, 2019.

[12] Gründl M. *Determinants of Physical Attractiveness: The Influence of Mediocrity, Symmetry and Sexual Dimorphism on the Attractiveness of Faces* [PhD dissertation]. Regensburg, Bavaria: Regensburg University; 2013.

[13] Grammer K, Thornhill R. Human (*Homo sapiens*) facial attractiveness and sexual selection: the role of symmetry and averageness. *J Comp Psych.* 1994;108:233–242.

[14] Rhodes G. The evolutionary psychology of facial beauty. *Annu Rev Psychol.* 2006;57:199–226.

[15] Ferrario V. Facial morphometry of television actresses compares with normal women. *J Oral Maxillofac Surg.* 1995;53:1008–1014.

[16] Tiddeman B, Burt DM, Perrett D. Computer graphics in facial perception research. *IEEE Computer Graphics and Applications.* Sept/Oct 2001;21(5):42–50.

[17] Tiddeman B, Perrett D. Transformation of dynamic facial image sequences using static 2D prototypes. *The Visual Computer.* June 2002;18(4):218–225.

[18] Chen J, Tiddeman B. Multi-cue facial feature detection and tracking under various illuminations. *Interntl J Robotics and Automation.* 2010;25(2):201.

[19] Perrett DI. Symmetry and human facial attractiveness. *Evol Hum Behav.* 1999;20(5):295–307.

[20] Rhodes G. Attractiveness of facial averageness and symmetry in non-western cultures: in search of biologically based standards of beauty. *Perception.* 2001;30:611–625.

[21] Rhodes G. Facial symmetry and the perception of beauty. *Psychonomic Bulletin & Review.* 1998; 5(4):659–669.

[22] Kowner, R. Facial asymmetry and attractiveness judgement in developmental perspective. *J Experimental Psychology: Human Perception and Performance.* 1996;22:662–675.

[23] Sutton, M. Lateral facial asymmetry: methods of assessment. *Angle Orthodontist.* 1968;38:82–92.

[24] Choi KY. Analysis of facial asymmetry. *Arch Craniofac Surg.* 2015;16(1):1–10.

[25] Langlois JH, Roggman LA, Musselman L. What is average and what is not average about attractive faces? *Psychol. Sci.* 1994 5:214.

[26] Korthase KM, Trenholme I. Perceived age and perceived physical attractiveness. *Percept Mot Skills.* 1982;54:1251–1258. doi: 10.2466/pms.1982.54.3c.1251

[27] Wernick M, Manaster GJ. Age and the perception of age and attractiveness. *The Gerontologist.* 1984;24:408–414. doi: 10.1093/geront/24.4.408

[28] Mathes EW, Brennan SM, Haugen PM, Rice HB. Ratings of physical attractiveness as a function of age. *J Soc Psychol.* 1985;125:157–168. doi: 10.1080/00224545.1985.9922868

[29] McLellan B, McKelvie SJ. Effects of age and gender on perceived facial attractiveness. *Can J Behav Sci.* 1993;25:135–142. doi: 10.1037/h0078790

[30] Henss R. Perceiving age and attractiveness in facial photographs. *J Appl Soc Psychol.* 1991;21:933–946. doi: 10.1111/j.1559-1816.1991.tb00451.x

[31] Maestripieri D, Klimczuk AC, Traficonte DM, Wilson MC. A greater decline in female facial attractiveness during middle age reflects women's loss of reproductive value. *Front Psychol.* February 28, 2014;5:179.

[32] Johnston VS, Solomon CJ, Gibson SJ, et al. Human facial beauty: current theories and methodologies. *Arch Facial Plast Surg.* 2003;5:371.

[33] Cunningham MR. Measuring the physical in physical attractiveness: quasi-experiments on the sociobiology of female facial beauty. *J Pers Soc Psychol.* 1986;50:925.

[34] Johnston VS, Franklin M. Is beauty in the eye of the beholder? *Ethol Sociobio.* 1993;14:183–9.

[35] Perrett DI, May KA, Yoshikawa S. Facial shape and judgments of female attractiveness. *Nature* 1994;368:239–242.

[36] Perrett DI, Lee KJ, Penton-Voak I, et al. Effects of sexual dimorphism on facial attractiveness. *Nature* 1998;394:884–887.

[37] Rhodes G, Hickford C, Jeffery L. Sextypicality and attractiveness: are supermale and superfemale faces super-attractive? *Br J Psychol.* 2000;91:125–140.

[38] Russell R. Sex, beauty, and the relative luminance of facial features. *Perception* 2003; 32:1093–107.

[39] Cunningham MR, Barbee AP, Pike CL. What do women want? Facialmetric assessment of multiple motives in the perception of male facial physical attractiveness. *J Personal Soc Psychol.* 1990;59:61–72.

[40] Gillen B. Physical attractiveness: a determinant of two types of goodness. *Personal Soc Psychol Bull.* 1981;7:384–387.

[41] Koehler N, Simmons LW, Rhodes G, Peters M. The relationship between sexual dimorphism in human faces and fluctuating asymmetry. *Proc R Soc Lond Ser B Biol Sci.* 2004;271:S233–S36.

[42] Neave N, Laing S, Fink B, Manning JT. Second to fourth digit ratio, testosterone and perceived male dominance. *Proc R Soc Lond Ser B Biol Sci.* 2003;270:2167–2172.

[43] Penton-Voak IS, Jacobson A, Trivers R. Populational differences in attractiveness judgments of male and female faces: comparing British and Jamaican samples. *Evol Hum Behav.* 2004;25:355–370.

[44] Levin EI. Dental esthetics and the golden proportion. *J Prosthet Dent.* 1978;40:244–252.

[45] Marquardt SR. Dr. Stephen R. Marquardt on the golden decagon and human facial beauty. Interview by Gottlieb. *J Clin Orthod.* 2002;36(6):339–347.

[46] Bashour M. An objective system for measuring facial attractiveness. *Plast Reconstr Surg.* 2006;118:757–774.

[47] Holland E. Marquardt's Phi mask: pitfalls of relying on fashion models and the golden ratio to describe a beautiful face. *Aesthetic Plast Surg.* March 2008;32(2):200–208. doi: 10.1007/s00266-007-9080-z

IMAGE CREDITS

© Andrew J. Hayduke, M.D.

Figures 30, 32, 34, 36, 37, 38, 39, 40, 41, 42, 43, 44, 45, 46, 47, 48, 49, 50, 51, 52, 53, 54, 55, 56, 57, 58, 59, 60, 61, 62, 63, 64, 65, 66, 67, 68, 69, 70, 71, 72, 73, 74, 75, 76, 77, 78, 79, 80, 81, 82, 83, 84, 85, 86, 87, 88, 89, 90, 91, 92, 93, 94, 95, 96, 97, 98, 99, 104, 105, 106, 107, 108, 113, 114, 115, 116, 117, 118, 119, 120, 121, 122, 123, 124, 125

© Martin Grundl

Figure 103

© Gillian Rhodes

Figures 109, 110

© F.L.C./ADAGP, Paris/Artists Rights Society (ARS), New York 2020

Figure 13

Courtesy of the Wikimedia Foundation

Figures 1, 2, 3, 4, 5, 6, 10, 15, 16, 17, 18, 19, 100,

Courtesy of the U.S. National Library of Medicine

Figures 101, 102

© Shutterstock

Figures 8, 9, 11, 12, 14, 29, 31, 33, 35, 112

© PictureLux/The Hollywood Archive/Alamy Stock Photo

Figure 111 (left image)

© Garcia/Gamma-Rapho/Getty Images

Figure 111 (middle image)

© Gilles Bassignac/Gamma-Rapho/Getty Images

Figure 111 (right image)

All golden ratio overlay grids and golden ratio labels applied to the images within this book are © Andrew J. Hayduke, M.D. (unless otherwise noted). Cover art and design © Andrew J. Hayduke, M.D.

INDEX

Page numbers with *f* and *t* indicate figures and tables, respectively.

I

J

K

L

M

ABOUT THE AUTHOR

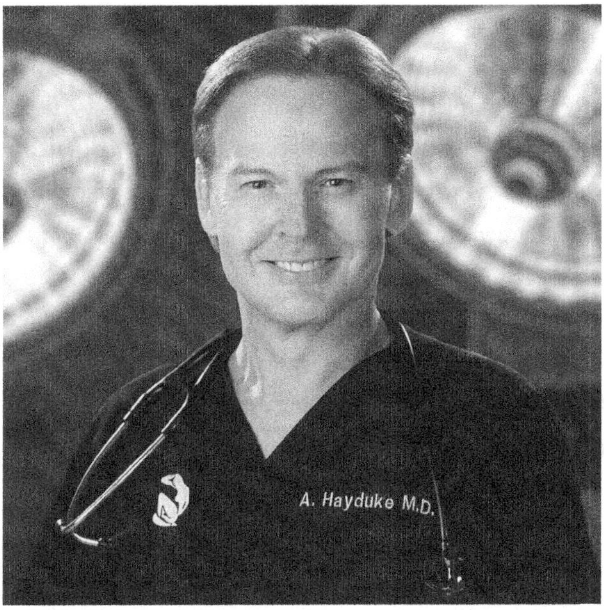

DR. ANDREW HAYDUKE

is a Beverly Hills plastic surgeon. Over several decades of practice, he has performed thousands upon thousands of plastic surgical procedures on the faces and breasts of clients from all over the world. He is the inventor of the innovative Divine Face® and Divine Breasts® analytical systems that scientifically evaluate the human face and breasts for anatomic beauty. He owns several US patents for his cutting-edge methodologies and is considered a pioneer in the field of anatomic beauty analysis.

Dr. Hayduke was chosen for the prestigious "Best Doctors" list by *U.S. News and World Report* and was featured in the national edition of *The New York Times* as one of the "Top Cosmetic Doctors in the Nation." He was chosen as a "Top Doctor" multiple times by *Palm Springs Life* magazine and was honored as one of the "Best of Beverly Hills" by the U.S. Commerce Association. He has served several terms as the Chief of Plastic Surgery of a Southern California medical center. Dr. Hayduke currently practices plastic surgery in Beverly Hills and Palm Springs, California. In his free time, he enjoys creating realistic figurative clay sculptures and playing guitar. He has a passion for endeavors that involve artistry, creativity, and the use of his hands.

DrHayduke.com

IVORY CROWN PRESS

Made in the USA
Las Vegas, NV
16 June 2026

48995821R00174